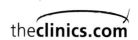

UROLOGIC CLINICS

OF NORTH AMERICA

Overactive Bladder

GUEST EDITOR
Michael B. Chancellor, MD

CONSULTING EDITOR
Martin I. Resnick, MD

November 2006 • Volume 33 • Number 4

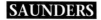

An Imprint of Elsevier, Inc.
PHILADELPHIA   LONDON   TORONTO   MONTREAL   SYDNEY   TOKYO

W.B. SAUNDERS COMPANY

A Division of Elsevier Inc.

1600 John F. Kennedy Boulevard • Suite 1800 • Philadelphia, Pennsylvania 19103-2899

http://www.theclinics.com

UROLOGIC CLINICS OF NORTH AMERICA	**Volume 33, Number 4**
November 2006	**ISSN 0094-0143**
Editor: Kerry Holland	**ISBN 1-4160-3920-1**

The ideas and opinions expressed in *Urologic Clinics of North America* do not necessarily reflect those of the Publisher. The Publisher does not assume any responsibility for any injury and/or damage to persons or property arising out of or related to any use of the material contained in this periodical. The reader is advised to check the appropriate medical literature and the product information currently provided by the manufacturer of each drug to be administered to verify the dosage, the method and duration of administration, or contraindications. It is the responsibility of the treating physician or other health care professional, relying on independent experience and knowledge of the patient, to determine drug dosages and the best treatment for the patient. Mention of any product in this issue should not be construed as endorsement by the contributors, editors, or the Publisher of the product or manufacturers' claims.

Urologic Clinics of North America (ISSN 0094-0143) is published quarterly by Elsevier Inc., 360 Park Avenue South, New York, NY 10010-1710. Months of issue are February, May, August, and November. Business and Editorial Offices: 1600 John F. Kennedy Blvd., Suite 1800, Philadelphia, PA 19103-2899. Customer Service Office: 6277 Sea Harbor Drive, Orlando, FL 32887-4800. Periodicals postage paid at New York, NY and additional mailing offices. Subscription prices are $231.00 per year (US individuals), $358.00 per year (US institutions), $264.00 per year (Canadian individuals), $429.00 per year (Canadian institutions), $308.00 per year (foreign individuals), and $429.00 per year (foreign institutions). Foreign air speed delivery is included in all *Clinics* subscription prices. All prices are subject to change without notice. **POSTMASTER:** Send address changes to *Urologic Clinics of North America*, Elsevier Periodicals Customer Service, 6277 Sea Harbor Drive, Orlando, FL 32887-4800. **Customer Service: 1-800-654-2452 (US). From outside the US, call 1-407-345-4000.**

Urologic Clinics of North America is covered in *Index Medicus*, *Excerpta Medica*, *Current Contents/ Clinical Medicine*, *Science Citation Index*, and *ISI/BIOMED*.

Printed in the United States of America.

GOAL STATEMENT

The goal of *Urologic Clinics of North America* is to keep practicing urologists and urology residents up to date with current clinical practice in urology by providing timely articles reviewing the state of the art in patient care.

ACCREDITATION

The Urologic Clinics of North America is planned and implemented in accordance with the Essential Areas and Policies of the Accreditation Council for Continuing Medical Education (ACCME) through the joint sponsorship of the University of Virginia School of Medicine and Elsevier. The University of Virginia School of Medicine is accredited by the ACCME to provide continuing medical education for physicians.

The University of Virginia School of Medicine designates this educational activity for a maximum of *15 AMA PRA Category 1 Credits™*. Physicians should only claim credit commensurate with the extent of their participation in the activity.

The American Medical Association has determined that physicians not licensed in the US who participate in this CME activity are eligible for *15 AMA PRA Category 1 Credits™*.

Credit can be earned by reading the text material, taking the CME examination online at http://www.theclinics.com/home/cme, and completing the evaluation. After taking the test, you will be required to review any and all incorrect answers. Following completion of the test and evaluation, your credit will be awarded and you may print your certificate.

FACULTY DISCLOSURE/CONFLICT OF INTEREST

The University of Virginia School of Medicine, as an ACCME accredited provider, endorses and strives to comply with the Accreditation Council for Continuing Medical Education (ACCME) Standards of Commercial Support, Commonwealth of Virginia statutes, University of Virginia policies and procedures, and associated federal and private regulations and guidelines on the need for disclosure and monitoring of proprietary and financial interests that may affect the scientific integrity and balance of content delivered in continuing medical education activities under our auspices.

The University of Virginia School of Medicine requires that all CME activities accredited through this institution be developed independently and be scientifically rigorous, balanced and objective in the presentation/discussion of its content, theories and practices.

All authors/editors participating in an accredited CME activity are expected to disclose to the readers relevant financial relationships with commercial entities occurring within the past 12 months (such as grants or research support, employee, consultant, stock holder, member of speakers bureau, etc.). The University of Virginia School of Medicine will employ appropriate mechanisms to resolve potential conflicts of interest to maintain the standards of fair and balanced education to the reader. Questions about specific strategies can be directed to the Office of Continuing Medical Education, University of Virginia School of Medicine, Charlottesville, Virginia.

The authors/editors listed below have identified no professional or financial affiliations for themselves or their spouse/partner:
Kerry Holland, Acquisitions Editor; Fernando De Miguel, PhD; Akira Furuta, MD; Michael Ingber, MD; Jamie A. Kanofsky, MD; Dae Kyung Kim, MD, PhD; Yong-Tae Kim, MD; Ji Youl Lee, MD; Wendy W. Leng, MD; Shelby Morrisroe, MD; Martin I. Resnick, MD (Consulting Editor); Jonathan S. Starkman, MD; Catherine A. Thomas, PhD; Shachi Tyagi, MD; and Osamu Yamaguchi, MD, PhD.

The authors/editors listed below identified the following professional or financial affiliations for themselves or their spouse/partner:
Michael Chancellor, MD (Guest Editor) is an independent contractor and a consultant for Pfizer, Alergen, Cook, Inc., and GlaxoSmithKline.
G. Willy Davila, MD is a consultant and on the speaker's bureau for Watson Pharmaceuticals
Ananias Diokno, MD is on the Advisory Committee/Board for Ortho-Urology; on the speaker's bureau for Astellas Pharma and Medtronic; and serves as an investigator for Eli-Lilly and GlaxoSmithKline.
Roger R. Dmochowski, MD is a consultant for Watson and Novartis.
Yukio Hayashi, PhD is employed by Taiho Pharmaceutical Co., Ltd.
Masahide Higaki, PhD is employed by Astellas Pharma, Inc.
Leaf Huang, PhD owns stock and is a patent holder for Lipella Pharmaceuticals.
Jon Kaufman, PhD, MBA is the president of Lipella Pharmaceuticals.
Karl J. Kreder, MD is on the speaker's bureau and Advisory Committee/Board, and serves as a consultant, for Astellas and Pfizer; owns stock in Merck, and is on the speaker's bureau for Merck.
Hitoshi Masuda, MD, PhD is a consultant for Indevus and Pfizer.
Victor W. Nitti, MD is on the speaker's bureau and Advisory Committee/Board for Novartis and Pfizer; is a consultant and is on the Advisory Committee/Board for Allergan; is an independent contractor and a consultant, and is on the speaker's bureau for Schwarz Pharma; is an independent contractor and is on the Advisory Committee/Board for Watson; and is on the Advisory Committee/Board for Astellas and Ortho McNeil.
Christopher Smith, MD is a consultant for, is on the Advisory Committee/Board of, and has a research contract with, Allergan, Inc.
David R. Staskin, MD is a consultant, serves on the Advisory Committee/Board, and is on the speakers' bureau for Indevus/Esprit, Pfizer, and Watson; serves on the Advisory Committee/Board and is on the speakers' bureau for Ortho-McNeil; is on the speakers' bureau for Novartis; and, serves on the Advisory Committee/Board for Astellas.
William Steers, MD is a consultant, serves on the Advisory Committee/Board, and is on the speakers' bureau for Pfizer, Novartis, and Astellas.
Pradeep Tyagi, PhD is a consultant for Lipella Pharmaceuticals.
Naoki Yoshimura, MD, PhD is a consultant for Indevus.

Disclosure of Discussion of non-FDA approved uses for pharmaceutical products and/or medical devices:
The University of Virginia School of Medicine, as an ACCME provider, requires that all faculty presenters identify and disclose any "off label" uses for pharmaceutical and medical device products. The University of Virginia School of Medicine recommends that each physician fully review all the available data on new products or procedures prior to instituting them with patients.

TO ENROLL

To enroll in the *Urologic Clinics of North America* Continuing Medical Education program, call customer service at 1-800-654-2452 or visit us online at www.theclinics.com/home/cme. The CME program is available to subscribers for an additional fee of $195.00.

CONSULTING EDITOR

MARTIN I. RESNICK, MD, Lester Persky Professor and Chairman, Department of Urology, Case Medical Center, Cleveland, Ohio

GUEST EDITOR

MICHAEL B. CHANCELLOR, MD, Professor, Department of Urology, University of Pittsburgh School of Medicine, Pittsburgh, Pennsylvania

CONTRIBUTORS

MICHAEL B. CHANCELLOR, MD, Professor, Department of Urology, University of Pittsburgh School of Medicine, Pittsburgh, Pennsylvania

G. WILLY DAVILA, MD, Chairman, Department of Gynecology, Head, Section of Urogynecology and Reconstructive Pelvic Surgery, Cleveland Clinic Florida, Weston, Florida

FERNANDO DE MIGUEL, PhD, Assistant Professor, Department of Urology, University of Pittsburgh School of Medicine, Pittsburgh, Pennsylvania

ANANIAS DIOKNO, MD, FACS, Peter & Florine Minestrelli Distinguished Chair in Urology, Department of Urology, William Beaumont Hospital, Royal Oak, Michigan

ROGER R. DMOCHOWSKI, MD, Professor of Urology, Department of Urologic Surgery, Vanderbilt University Medical Center, Nashville, Tennessee

AKIRA FURUTA, MD, Postdoctoral Associate, Department of Urology, University of Pittsburgh School of Medicine, Pittsburgh, Pennsylvania

YUKIO HAYASHI, PhD, Taiho Pharmaceutical Company, Tokyo, Japan

MASAHIDE HIGAKI, PhD, Postdoctoral Associate, Department of Urology, University of Pittsburgh School of Medicine, Pittsburgh, Pennsylvania

LEAF HUANG, PhD, School of Pharmacy, University of North Carolina at Chapel Hill, Chapel Hill, North Carolina

MICHAEL INGBER, MD, Urology Resident, Department of Urology, William Beaumont Hospital, Royal Oak, Michigan

JAMIE A. KANOFSKY, MD, Resident, Department of Urology, New York University School of Medicine, New York, New York

JONATHAN KAUFMAN, PhD, MBA, Lipella Pharmaceuticals, Pittsburgh, Pennsylvania

DAE KYUNG KIM, MD, PhD, Assistant Professor, Department of Urology, Eulji University School of Medicine, Daejeon, Korea

YONG-TAE KIM, MD, Associate Professor, College of Medicine, Hanyang University, Seoul, South Korea

KARL J. KREDER, MD, Professor and Clinical Vice Chair, Director of Female Urology and Urodynamics, Department of Urology, University of Iowa, Iowa City, Iowa

JI YOUL LEE, MD, Department of Urology, Catholic University of Korea, School of Medicine, Seoul, Korea

WENDY W. LENG, MD, Assistant Professor, Department of Urology, University of Pittsburgh School of Medicine, Pittsburgh, Pennsylvania

HITOSHI MASUDA, MD, PhD, Associate Professor, Department of Urology and Reproductive Medicine, Graduate School, Tokyo Medical and Dental University, Tokyo, Japan

SHELBY N. MORRISROE, MD, Department of Urology, University of Pittsburgh School of Medicine, Pittsburgh, Pennsylvania

VICTOR W. NITTI, MD, FACS, Associate Professor and Vice Chairman, Department of Urology, New York University School of Medicine, New York, New York

CHRISTOPHER SMITH, MD, Department of Urology, University of Pittsburgh School of Medicine, Pittsburgh, Pennsylvania

JONATHAN S. STARKMAN, MD, Clinical Instructor, Department of Urologic Surgery, Vanderbilt University Medical Center, Nashville, Tennessee

DAVID R. STASKIN, MD, Associate Professor, Department of Urology, New York Presbyterian Hospital, Weill-Cornell Medical College, New York, New York

WILLIAM D. STEERS, MD, FACS, Hovey Dabney Professor and Chair, Department of Urology, University of Virginia School of Medicine, University of Virginia Health System, Charlottesville, Virginia

CATHERINE A. THOMAS, PhD, Postdoctoral Associate, Department of Urology, University of Pittsburgh School of Medicine, Pittsburgh, Pennsylvania

PRADEEP TYAGI, PhD, Department of Urology, University of Pittsburgh School of Medicine; and Department of Urology, Montefiore Hospital, Pittsburgh, Pennsylvania

SHACHI TYAGI, MD, Postdoctoral Associate, Department of Urology, University of Pittsburgh School of Medicine, Pittsburgh, Pennsylvania

OSAMU YAMAGUCHI, MD, PhD, Professor, Department of Urology, Fukushima Medical University School of Medicine, Fukushima City, Fukushima, Japan

NAOKI YOSHIMURA, MD, PhD, Associate Professor, Department of Urology, University of Pittsburgh School of Medicine, Pittsburgh, Pennsylvania

CONTENTS

> The International Continence Society recognizes the overactive bladder (OAB) as a "symptom syndrome suggestive of lower urinary tract dysfunction" that is defined as "urgency, with or without urge incontinence, usually with frequency and nocturia." Patients who have OAB are often sleep deprived and their sexual life is hindered. These patients have a restricted social life and an increased risk for depression. Accurate prevalence figures are difficult to obtain because most patients consider OAB an inevitable part of aging and some patients are too embarrassed to seek diagnosis. Primary care physicians need to be educated about the importance of identifying this clinical problem and managing it in a way that will minimize morbidity and maximize quality-of-life improvement. This article describes the various aspects of OAB, with special emphasis on epidemiology and morbidity.

CURRENT THERAPY: WHAT IS SPECIAL ABOUT EACH DRUG?

> Oxybutynin has been used for the management of detrusor overactivity for over 30 years and has withstood medical scrutiny and the test of time throughout the world. Although several agents in the class of bladder relaxants have only recently been studied, oxybutynin's effectiveness in reducing urinary frequency and urge urinary incontinence is unquestioned in the medical literature. Oxybutynin is extremely safe and effective in almost every population including children, the elderly, and those who have neurogenic bladder. With more preparations available and more dosing flexibility than any other anticholinergic medication on the market, oxybutynin remains the "gold standard" for first-line therapy for patients who have detrusor overactivity.

WHAT CAN UROLOGISTS DO FOR REFRACTORY OVERACTIVE BLADDER?

WHAT IS NEW IN OVERACTIVE BLADDER SCIENCE?

Interactions between muscarinic receptors in the urothelium, afferent nerves, or myofibroblasts and locally released acetylcholine might be involved in the emergence of detrusor overactivity and OAB. Therefore, antimuscarinic agents may be effective in treating OAB not only by suppression of muscarinic receptor-mediated detrusor muscle contractions but also by modulation of muscarinic receptor-bladder afferent interactions.

FORTHCOMING ISSUES

RECENT ISSUES

ELSEVIER
SAUNDERS

Urol Clin N Am 33 (2006) xiii

UROLOGIC
CLINICS
of North America

Foreword

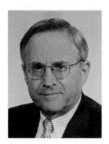

Martin I. Resnick, MD
Consulting Editor

We hear about it every day, whether it is on a television commercial, in a newspaper advertisement, or a symptom reported by one of our patients. Overactive bladder is not only a common problem but also one of which our patient population is well aware. It is more common in women, and not only is it responsible for impacting on the lifestyle of the affected patient but it can also lead to a reclusive lifestyle and, at times, the need for assisted living care because of urinary incontinence and associated embarrassment. The cost to the patient and society is significant.

In this issue of the *Urologic Clinics of North America*, Dr. Michael Chancellor with the assistance of multiple authors has reviewed the salient aspects of this disorder. The epidemiology, morbidity, and associated economic and social issues are fully addressed. In addition, the various medications that are available are reviewed; similarities and differences are noted. Newer approaches such as sacral nerve stimulation and the application of bladder toxic agents are also discussed in a logical manner so that these newer techniques are placed in context with more standard therapy. Finally, new pharmaceuticals such as β_3-adrenergic receptor agonists are also reviewed.

This issue should be of interest not only to all urologists caring for patients who have overactive bladder but also to all physicians caring for these patients, whether they be gynecologists, internists, or family physicians.

Martin I. Resnick, MD
Department of Urology
Case Medical Center
Cleveland, OH, USA

E-mail address: martin.resnick@case.edu

ELSEVIER
SAUNDERS

Urol Clin N Am 33 (2006) xv–xvi

UROLOGIC
CLINICS
of North America

Preface

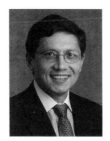

Michael B. Chancellor, MD
Guest Editor

Overactive bladder (OAB) is a highly prevalent disorder that affects the lives of millions of people worldwide. With a large population of the baby-boomer generation aging rapidly, it will become increasingly important to improve primary care physicians' awareness of this important problem. Only with awareness can patient quality-of-life improvement be maximized while minimizing morbidity of OAB.

OAB is a symptom syndrome suggestive of lower urinary tract dysfunction by the International Continence Society (ICS). It is a common and important medical problem faced by the health care community worldwide. It has been reported that the total costs of urinary incontinence in the United States in 2000 were over $26 billion. Of this amount, direct costs accounted for $25.6 billion and indirect costs accounted for $700 million.

The median prevalence of incontinence in women varies from 14% to 40.5% (23.5% using the ICS definition). In men, the prevalence of incontinence varies from 4.6% to 15%. In women, urge and mixed incontinence account for a median relative share of 51% of cases, whereas in men, the combined total is 92%. Approximately 33% of patients who have OAB have urinary urge incontinence. The remaining patients do not, complaining only of urgency, generally with frequency and nocturia.

Responses by country vary somewhat. The prevalence percentages of OAB for men and women in Spain were reported as 20% and 24%, respectively, whereas for men and women in France, they were 11% and 13%, respectively. In all, 79% of these patients have had their symptoms for 1 year or more, and 49% have had them for more than 3 years. Of those who have bladder symptoms, frequency is the most commonly reported symptom (85%), followed by urgency (54%) and urge incontinence (36%).

The prevalence of OAB and of all three symptoms increases with advancing age. This trend is apparent in men and in women. For men and women, respectively, prevalence percentages for OAB have been reported as follows: 3.4% and 8.7% for those 40 to 44 years old, 9.8% and 11.9% for those 50 to 54 years old, 18.9% and 16.9% for those 60 to 64 years old, 22.3% and 22.1% for those 70 to 74 years old, and 41.9% and 31.3% for those 75 or more years old.

The slope for the increase in prevalence of OAB in men and women with respect to age is approximately the same. The prevalence of OAB "dry" seems to level off in men at about age 60 years and in women at about age 50 years. The prevalence of OAB "wet" is low in men (3%) until about age 60 years, and this number increases to approximately 8% at age 65 years or older, whereas for women, the prevalence increases from approximately 12% at age 60 years to approximately 20% at age 65 years or older.

One of the most important concerns of all physicians is that poor bladder control can cause complications and result in falls and fractures. A recent prospective study found that the economic and clinical impact of OAB is not limited to the disease itself because OAB patients in a managed care setting also had increased medical costs associated with related comorbidities. The mean annual medical charges of 11,556 patients of OAB (≥18 years old) obtained from submitted insurance claims were significantly higher than those of 11,556 matched control subjects who did not have OAB. A significantly higher prevalence of all comorbid conditions including depression, skin infections, and vulvovaginitis was seen in patients who had OAB compared with control subjects.

It has also been reported that urinary incontinence is independently associated with falls and fractures among community-dwelling elderly women. Women who have weekly urge incontinence have a 26% greater risk of sustaining a fall and a 34% increased risk of fracture after adjusting for other causes. More frequent incontinence has been associated with increased risk, and women who have daily urge incontinence have a 35% and 45% increased risk of sustaining falls and fractures, respectively.

There is an association between depression and urge incontinence. The prevalence of depression is 60% in those who have idiopathic urge incontinence, 42% in patients who have mixed incontinence, and only 14% in patients who have stress incontinence.

Urinary tract infections and skin infections are factors that increase the cost of OAB; however, there is a potential reduction in health care costs for patients who receive treatment for OAB. It has been shown that after the diagnosis of OAB, the number of services received for urinary tract infections and skin infections decreases 40% and 60%, respectively.

Two thirds of men and women who have OAB report that their symptoms have an effect on daily living. Frequency and urgency alone are almost as common as urge incontinence as reasons for seeking help. OAB also affects sexual function. Recent studies have shown that urinary incontinence significantly reduces sexual function in premenopausal sexually active women.

Without fail, in all epidemiologic studies, more than 80% of the women responding have reported that their symptoms of urinary incontinence symptoms are a cause of concern. An increase in the severity of incontinence correlated with a negative impact on quality of life characterized by low self-esteem and reduced social life. The most common reactions to the urinary incontinence component of OAB were embarrassment, frustration, anxiety, annoyance, depression, and fear of odor.

I think you will enjoy reading this issue of the *Urology Clinics of North America*. The best of the best authorities have contributed articles that highlight their known clinical expertise. In addition, we have contributions from leading translational scientists that offer urologists a perspective on new approaches that may be used to treat OAB over the next 2 decades. Finally, I would like to thank Dr. Resnick for the opportunity to be the Guest Editor. He has allowed me the freedom to "push the envelope" on putting together a state-of-the-art issue on OAB and, at the same time, offered his experience and wisdom on editing a successful Clinics issue of which I am very proud. Thank you Marty.

Michael B. Chancellor, MD
Department of Urology
University of Pittsburgh School of Medicine
Suite 700, Kaufmann Building
3471 Fifth Avenue
Pittsburgh, PA 15213, USA

E-mail address: chancellormb@upmc.edu

ELSEVIER
SAUNDERS

Urol Clin N Am 33 (2006) 433–438

UROLOGIC
CLINICS
of North America

The Overactive Bladder: Epidemiology and Morbidity

Shachi Tyagi, MD[a], Catherine A. Thomas, PhD[a],
Yukio Hayashi, PhD[b], Michael B. Chancellor, MD[a],*

[a]*Department of Urology, University of Pittsburgh School of Medicine, Suite 700,
3471 Fifth Avenue, Pittsburgh, PA 15213, USA*
[b]*Taiho Pharmaceutical Company, Tokyo, Japan*

Overactive bladder (OAB), is defined by the International Continence Society (ICS), as a symptom syndrome suggestive of lower urinary tract dysfunction [1]. It is a common and important medical problem faced by the health care community worldwide. Wagner and Hu [2] reported that the total costs of urinary incontinence in the United States in 2000 were over $26 billion. Of this amount, direct costs accounted for $25.6 billion and indirect costs accounted for $700 million. It is unfortunate that we do not have a good cost analysis for patients who have OAB, including those who have "OAB wet" (OAB patients who have urge incontinence) and "OAB dry" (OAB patients who do not have urge incontinence). Hu and Wagner [3] noted that it is possible that the economic burden of OAB is even greater than that of urinary incontinence.

Overactive bladder epidemiology

The median prevalence of incontinence in women has been reported as varying from 14% to 40.5% (23.5% using the ICS definition). In men, the prevalence of incontinence has varied from 4.6% to 15%. In women, urge and mixed incontinence accounted for a median relative share of 51% of cases, whereas in men, the combined total was 92% [4,5]. Approximately 33% of patients who had OAB had urinary urge incontinence. The remaining patients did not, complaining only of urgency, generally with

frequency and nocturia [4,5]. Milsom and colleagues [6] reported on a study performed by the Svenska Institute for Opinionsundersokingar/Gallup Network in France, Germany, Italy, Spain, Sweden, and the United Kingdom. This study used a telephone questionnaire involving a two-stage screening procedure, which first identified individuals who had bladder control problems and then characterized the nature of the urinary condition. The first step specifically excluded individuals whose only complaint was urinary tract infection. Symptoms attributable to OAB were identified by positive response to specific questions on frequency, urgency, and urge incontinence. Frequency caused by OAB was arbitrarily defined as greater than eight micturitions in 24 hours. For nocturia, the working definition specified that patients had to get up two or more times a night to urinate. Respondents could have greater than one OAB symptom but were classified only once as having OAB. Currently, OAB is further classified into two groups: OAB wet and OAB dry [7].

Positive responses in this study [6] that were suggestive only of stress incontinence, prostatic obstruction, or the occurrence of urinary tract infection resulted in exclusion from further investigation. Respondents who were 40 or more years old and had OAB only or mixed symptoms were included. The interviewed population totaled 16,776 subjects. Approximately 19% of all respondents reported current bladder symptoms, but overall, 16.6% of total respondents, 15.6% of men, and 17.4% of women reported symptoms suggestive of OAB.

Responses by country varied somewhat: the prevalence percentages of OAB for men and women in Spain were 20% and 24%, respectively,

---

* Corresponding author.
E-mail address: chancellormb@upmc.edu
(M.B. Chancellor).

whereas for men and women in France, they were 11% and 13%, respectively. In all, 79% of these patients had had their symptoms for 1 year or more, and 49% had had them for more than 3 years. Of the subjects who had bladder symptoms, frequency was the most commonly reported symptom (85%), followed by urgency (54%) and urge incontinence (36%).

The prevalence of OAB and of all three symptoms increased with advancing age. This trend was apparent in men and in women. For men and women, respectively, prevalence percentages of OAB were as follows: 3.4% and 8.7% for those 40 to 44 years old, 9.8% and 11.9% for those 50 to 54 years old, 18.9% and 16.9% for those 60 to 64 years old, 22.3% and 22.1% for those 70 to 74 years old, and 41.9% and 31.3% for those 75 or more years old.

The National Overactive Bladder Evaluation study

The National Overactive Bladder Evaluation (NOBLE) study was conducted to provide a clinically valid research definition of OAB [8]. The NOBLE study also estimated OAB overall prevalence and the individual burden of illness and explored differences between OAB populations (ie, those who are incontinent and those who are dry) [2,8]. A computer-assisted telephone interview was developed to estimate variation and prevalence of OAB by demographic and other factors. This telephone interview was assessed for reliability and clinical validity. Clinical validity was assessed by comparison with a clinician's diagnosis. The sensitivity and the specificity of the computer-assisted telephone interview for OAB were 61% and 91%, respectively.

The validated United States national telephone survey involved 5204 adults (≥ 18 years old) who were representative of the noninstitutionalized United States population with respect to sex, age, and geographic region. OAB dry was defined as four or more episodes of urgency in the previous 4 weeks, with frequency of greater than eight times per day or the use of one or more coping behaviors to control bladder function. OAB wet included the same criteria as OAB dry in addition to three or more episodes of urinary incontinence in the previous 4 weeks that were clearly not episodes of stress incontinence. The overall prevalence of OAB was reported as 16.9% in women and 16.2% in men, increasing with age. The overall prevalence percentages of OAB dry

and OAB wet in women were 7.6% and 9.3%, respectively, whereas in men, they were 13.6% and 2.6%, respectively. In the United States, these figures translate to 33.3 million adults who have OAB, 12.2 million who have incontinence and 21.2 million who do not.

The slope for the increase in prevalence of OAB in men and women with respect to age was approximately same. The prevalence of OAB dry seemed to level off in men at about age 60 years and in women at about age 50 years. The prevalence of OAB wet was low in men (3%) until about age 60 years, and this number increased to approximately 8% at age 65 years or older, whereas for women, the prevalence increased from approximately 12% at age 60 years to approximately 20% at age 65 years or older.

Morbidity of overactive bladder

One of the most important concerns of all physicians is that poor bladder control can cause complications and result in falls and fractures [9,10]. Table 1 lists the top 12 reasons why women who have OAB seek treatment. Table 2 lists other medical conditions associated with OAB. A recent prospective study found that the economic and clinical impact of OAB is not limited to the disease itself because OAB patients in a managed care setting also had increased medical costs associated with related comorbidities [11]. The mean annual medical charges of 11,556 patients of OAB (≥ 18 years old) obtained from submitted insurance claims were significantly higher than those of 11,556 matched control subjects who did not have OAB [11]. A significantly higher prevalence of all comorbid conditions including depression, skin infections, and vulvovaginitis was seen in patients who had OAB compared with control subjects.

Brown and colleagues [12] also reported that urinary incontinence is independently associated with falls and fractures among community-dwelling elderly women. Women who have weekly urge incontinence have a 26% greater risk of sustaining a fall and a 34% increased risk of fracture after adjusting for other causes. More frequent incontinence was associated with increased risk, and women who had daily urge incontinence had a 35% and 45% increased risk of sustaining falls and fractures, respectively.

There is an association between depression and urge incontinence in a survey that used a Beck Depression Inventory [12]. The prevalence of

Table 1

Top dozen reasons why women with overactive bladder seek treatment

Reasons for seeking treatment	Most important reason (n = 605) (%)	All that apply (n = 754) (%)
Concern that condition would get worse	20.5	168.4
Had to start wearing panty liners/pads	4.3	156.5
Concern that condition was not normal	12.4	154.0
Increasing concern about possibility of an embarrassing accident	7.6	146.0
Concern that leakage or urine loss was a symptom of a more serious condition	14.7	241.9
Interference with daily activities	6.6	41.4
Worry that others could smell the odor caused by leakage or involuntary loss of urine	8.8	41.3
Interference with physical activities	5.6	39.3
Frequency of leakage or urine loss increased	3.5	32.8
An embarrassing accident occurred	3.3	24.8
Interference with work activities	0.8	24.7
The amount of leakage or urine loss increased	2.3	23.7

Data from Coyne KS, et al. The impact of urinary urgency and frequency on health-related quality of life in overactive bladder: results from a national community surrey. Value Health 2004;7(4):455–63.

depression was 60% in those who had idiopathic urge incontinence, 42% in patients who had mixed incontinence, and only 14% in patients who had stress incontinence. The extent to which OAB alone contributes to sleep disturbances remains unclear because many individuals, particularly elderly individuals, report sleep problems that are unrelated to the nocturia component of OAB. Brown and colleagues [12] also noted that because previous studies have demonstrated that urge incontinence has been associated with frequency/urgency and nocturia, OAB symptom, and not just urge incontinence, has the potential to increase the risk of falls and fractures among elderly women.

Urinary tract infections and skin infections are factors that increase the cost of OAB. There is a potential reduction in health care costs for patients receiving treatment for OAB. A recent report on pharmaceutic outcomes from a study involving 2496 chronic OAB patients enrolled in the California Medicaid (Medi-Cal) program showed that discontinuation of OAB treatment for more than 30 days increased the risk of urinary tract infection diagnosis by 37%, but other OAB/urinary incontinence–related comorbidities were not significantly affected [13]. A previous study on patients from the Medi-Cal program also reported that after the diagnosis of OAB, the number of services received for urinary tract infections and skin infections decreased 40% and 60%, respectively, and this decrease was associated with potential cost savings, sampling from the 1996 to 1997 Medi-Cal program [12].

Table 2

Other reported medical conditions associated with overactive bladder

Condition	No. of Continent OAB patients (%) (n = 228)	No. of Incontinent OAB patients (%) (n = 168)	No. of Control subject (%) (n = 523)	P
Diabetes	21 (9.3)	34 (20.4)	34 (6.5)	< 0.0001
Self = reported history of bladder surgery	36 (15.9)	36 (21.4)	10 (1.9)	< 0.0001
Self = reported prostate problems (n = 361)	32 (22.1)	21 (53.9)	26 (14.7)	< 0.0001
Interstitial cystitis	5 (2.2)	7 (4.2)	5 (1.0)	0.02
Central nervous system disorder	10 (4.4)	13 (7.7)	6 (1.2)	< 0.0001

Data from Teleman PM, et al. Overactive bladder: prevalence, risk factors and relation to stress incontinence in middle-aged women. Br Jobstet Gynaecol 2004;111(6):600–4.

Quality-of-life issues in overactive bladder

Up to 65% of men and 67% of women who had OAB reported that their symptoms had an effect on daily living [6]. Sixty percent of those who had symptoms found them bothersome enough to consult a medical practitioner. Frequency and urgency alone (59%) were almost as common as urge incontinence (66%) as reasons for seeking help. The cardinal symptoms of OAB are now considered to be urgency, frequency, and nocturia. In fact, urgency has been found to be significantly related to patients' quality of life [14,15].

Of those who sought medical care, only 27% were receiving medication for symptoms at the time of the interview [6]. Of those who were not taking medication, 27% had previously tried pharmacologic treatment (which had failed). Of those who were not taking medication and had never tried pharmacologic treatment, 54% reported that they would likely discuss the problem with a physician again and 46% would not. Of those in whom medication had failed, 65% reported that they would likely discuss the problem with a physician again and 35% would not.

In a study by Stewart and colleagues [16], illness impact was assessed by completed self-administered questionnaires on quality of life, depression status, and sleep quality. Quality of life was assessed with the 36-Item Short-Form (SF-36) Health Survey, a standardized generic instrument that measures health-related quality of life (HRQOL) during the previous month in eight domains (physical functioning, role functioning, social functioning, mental health, vitality, health perception, emotional role, and bodily pain). Depression status was assessed by the Center for Epidemiologic Studies Depression Scale, which is a self-reported scale developed to identify depression-related symptoms. Sleep quality was assessed by the Medical Outcomes Sleep Scale, a 12-item questionnaire that measures sleep disturbance, insomnia, sleep quality and duration, and restfulness. After adjusting for differences in comorbid illnesses and other demographic factors, men and women who had OAB wet and OAB dry had clinically and significantly lower quality-of-life subscores, more depression-related symptoms, and a poorer quality of sleep. A recent study studied the impact of urinary incontinence on sexual function in female patients [17].

Recently, studies have been done to assess the affect of OAB on sexual function. Kim and colleagues [18] enrolled 3372 women aged 20 to 49 years by way of a multicenter Internet survey and investigated their lower urinary tract symptoms and sexual activities using a structured questionnaire. OAB syndrome was detected in 12.7% of enrolled women, and this group had greater deterioration in sexual activity. In a different study, the Female Sexual Function Index (FSFI) was used to evaluate sexual function in 21 premenopausal incontinent women. The mean FSFI domain scores for desire, arousal, lubrication, orgasm, satisfaction, and pain of incontinent women were compared against 18 nearly age–matched healthy continent women. Except for pain, all of the domain scores were significantly lower in incontinent women than in healthy women, suggesting that urinary incontinence significantly reduces sexual functions in premenopausal sexually active women [17].

Liberman and colleagues [19] assessed the impact of symptoms of OAB on the quality of life in a community-based United States sample population. The survey was conducted in two phases: (1) a cross-sectional household telephone survey was performed among an age-stratified sample of 4896 adults; and (2) a follow-up questionnaire was mailed to a subset of these respondents to assess their HRQOL. The Medical Outcomes Study Short-Form 20 was used, which measures HRQOL during the previous month in six domains: physical functioning, role functioning, social functioning, mental health, health perception, and bodily pain. Both groups (OAB wet and OAB dry) had significantly lower crude HRQOL scores than the control groups in every domain.

Statistically significant differences were observed in five of the six domains for the total OAB group, in all six domains for the OAB wet group, and in three of the six domains for the OAB dry group. In the OAB dry group, after adjustment for confounders, individuals who had symptoms of frequency and urgency scored statistically significantly lower than the controls in all six HRQOL domains [19]. There were numeric differences for the frequency-only and urgency-only subgroups, but these did not reach statistical significance. Individuals reporting 11 or more micturitions per day had statistically significantly lower domain-specific scores than those of controls in the areas of physical functioning, mental health, and bodily pain. The HRQOL scores for individuals who had 9 to 10 micturitions per day were not significantly different from those of controls. Kobelt [20] reported the results of an assessment of HRQOL using the SF-36 in a Swedish population with established urge or mixed incontinence and indicated that this cohort scored significantly lower in all domains than the general Swedish population, matched for age and sex distribution. In addition, Kobelt [20] reported that to some extent, these results were confirmed using data from a clinical trial in the United States and Canada in which two treatments for urinary incontinence were compared with placebo.

The SF-36 scores of the trial population at baseline were significantly lower than those of the healthy, age-matched population in six of the eight domains [12]. In three of these domains (social functioning, role limitations caused by emotional problems, and mental health), the scores were significantly correlated with micturitions and leaks at baseline, whereas the correlations with scores in the domains of vitality and general health were of borderline significance. In a recent European study, a detailed questionnaire was mailed to 2960 women randomly selected from an earlier survey of 29,500 representative households in four countries (France, Germany, Spain and the United Kingdom) to assess the burden from urinary incontinence and its affect on quality of life. More than 80% of the women responding to the questionnaire reported that their symptoms of urinary incontinence symptoms were a cause of concern [21]. An increase in severity of incontinence correlated with a negative impact on quality of life characterized by low self-esteem and reduced social life [21]. A similar study was done in a United States population of 1046 women who self-reported symptoms of urinary incontinence. Most women completing the survey by way of electronic mail rated urinary symptoms as moderately or extremely annoying [22].

Abrams and colleagues [23] reported that patients who had OAB had a lower quality of life in the social and functional domains of the SF-36 compared with patients who had diabetes. They pointed out that many patients who have OAB tend to stop pursuing enjoyable social and physical activities, living with the condition in silence because they are too embarrassed to talk about their condition or are unaware that it can be treated. The most common reactions to the urinary incontinence component of OAB were embarrassment, frustration, anxiety, annoyance, depression, and fear of odor. Kelleher and colleagues [24] reported assessment of quality of life in OAB using the King's Health Questionnaire, a survey originally developed to evaluate quality of life in women who had urinary incontinence.

Using this survey, women who had OAB and incontinence were reported to have significantly greater quality-of-life impairment compared with women who had stress incontinence and normal urodynamic function [24]. A recently published report assessed the merits of a patient-reported outcome measure specific to stress, urge, and mixed urinary incontinence—the incontinence-specific quality of life (I-QOL) measure—in community studies and clinical trials with varying types and severity of urinary incontinence. The I-QOL is a reliable and valid measure of HRQOL, suitable for use in a variety of international settings.

These studies emphasize the difficulty in assessing impairment of quality of life in patients who have OAB [25]. Most of the studies assessed patients who had OAB wet. Impairment in this group is most likely greater than it is in the OAB dry group. Studies are underway to overcome the deficit in data on quality of life as it applies to the total OAB population and its subdivisions of OAB wet and OAB dry.

Summary

OAB is a highly prevalent disorder that affects the lives of millions of people worldwide. With a large population of the baby-boomer generation aging rapidly, it will become increasingly important to improve primary care physicians' awareness of this important problem. Only with awareness can patient quality-of-life improvement be maximized while minimizing morbidity of OAB.

References

[1] Wein AJ, Rovner ES. Definition and epidemiology of overactive bladder. Urology 2002;60(5 Suppl. 1): 7–12 [discussion: 12].

[2] Wagner TH, et al. Health-related consequences of overactive bladder. Am J Manag Care 2002;8(19 Suppl):S598–607.

[3] Hu TW, et al. Costs of urinary incontinence and overactive bladder in the United States: a comparative study. Urology 2004;63(3):461–5.

[4] Hampel C, et al. [Epidemiology and etiology of overactive bladder]. Urologe A 2003;42(6):776–86 [German].

[5] Milsom I, Stewart W, Thuroff J. The prevalence of overactive bladder. Am J Manag Care 2000;6(11 Suppl):S565–73.

[6] Milsom I, et al. How widespread are the symptoms of an overactive bladder and how are they managed? A population-based prevalence study. BJU Int 2001; 87(9):760–6.

[7] Tubaro A. Defining overactive bladder: epidemiology and burden of disease. Urology 2004;64(6 Suppl. 1): 2–6.

[8] Coyne KS, et al. The impact of urinary urgency and frequency on health-related quality of life in overactive bladder: results from a national community survey. Value Health 2004;7(4):455–63.

[9] Teleman PM, et al. Overactive bladder: prevalence, risk factors and relation to stress incontinence in middle-aged women. Br J Obstet Gynaecol 2004; 111(6):600–4.

[10] Asplund R. Nocturia in relation to sleep, health, and medical treatment in the elderly. BJU Int 2005; 96(Suppl 1):15–21.

[11] Darkow T, Fontes CL, Williamson TE. Costs associated with the management of overactive bladder and related comorbidities. Pharmacotherapy 2005; 25(4):511–9.

[12] Brown JS, McGhan WF, Chokroverty S. Comorbidities associated with overactive bladder. Am J Manag Care 2000;6(11 Suppl):S574–9.

[13] Yu YF, et al. Persistence and adherence of medications for chronic overactive bladder/urinary incontinence in the California Medicaid program. Value Health 2005;8(4):495–505.

[14] Tubaro A, Palleschi G. Overactive bladder: epidemiology and social impact. Curr Opin Obstet Gynecol 2005;17(5):507–11.

[15] Abrams P. Urgency: the key to defining the overactive bladder. BJU Int 2005;96(Suppl 1):1–3.

[16] Stewart WF, et al. Prevalence and burden of overactive bladder in the United States. World J Urol 2003; 20(6):327–36.

[17] Aslan G, et al. Sexual function in women with urinary incontinence. Int J Impot Res 2005;17(3): 248–51.

[18] Kim YH, Seo JT, Yoon H. The effect of overactive bladder syndrome on the sexual quality of life in Korean young and middle aged women. Int J Impot Res 2005;17(2):158–63.

[19] Liberman JN, et al. Health-related quality of life among adults with symptoms of overactive bladder: results from a US community-based survey. Urology 2001;57(6):1044–50.

[20] Kobelt G. Economic considerations and outcome measurement in urge incontinence. Urology 1997; 50(6A Suppl):100–7 [discussion: 108–10].

[21] Papanicolaou S, et al. Assessment of bothersomeness and impact on quality of life of urinary incontinence in women in France, Germany, Spain and the UK. BJU Int 2005;96(6):831–8.

[22] MacDiarmid S, Rosenberg M. Overactive bladder in women: symptom impact and treatment expectations. Curr Med Res Opin 2005;21(9): 1413–21.

[23] Abrams P, et al. Overactive bladder significantly affects quality of life. Am J Manag Care 2000;6(11 Suppl):S580–90.

[24] Kelleher CJ, et al. A new questionnaire to assess the quality of life of urinary incontinent women. Br J Obstet Gynaecol 1997;104(12):1374–9.

[25] Ross S, et al. Incontinence-specific quality of life measures used in trials of treatments for female urinary incontinence: a systematic review. Int Urogynecol J Pelvic Floor Dysfunct 2006;17(3): 272–85.

ELSEVIER
SAUNDERS

Urol Clin N Am 33 (2006) 439–445

UROLOGIC
CLINICS
of North America

Oxybutynin in Detrusor Overactivity

Ananias Diokno, MD, FACS*, Michael Ingber, MD

Department of Urology, William Beaumont Hospital, 3535 W. Thirteen Mile Road,
Suite 438, Royal Oak, MI 48073, USA

Oxybutynin clearly represents a special drug in its class of bladder relaxants. Although several alternative agents have only recently been studied, oxybutynin has been in existence for the management of detrusor overactivity for over 30 years. It has withstood medical scrutiny and the test of time throughout the world. Its effectiveness in reducing urinary frequency and urge urinary incontinence is unquestioned in the medical literature. Oxybutynin has been demonstrated urodynamically to increase bladder capacity and to blunt, if not abolish, detrusor overactivity. The drug is applicable for adults and pediatric patients 6 years and older. In addition, oxybutynin offers flexibility because of its extensive formulations including immediate-release forms and extended-release forms and dose formulations of 5, 10, and 15 mg. Its proven safety and tolerability have been based not only on randomized clinical trials but also, more effectively, on over 30 years of experience.

Background

Oxybutynin chloride has a long history of safety and efficacy dating back to the mid-1960s, when it was originally approved for the management of detrusor hyper-reflexia secondary to neurogenic bladder dysfunction. Originally developed by Majewski [1], oxybutynin was patented in 1965. Oxybutynin has both musculotropic relaxant activity and local anesthetic activity, and has been one of the most extensively studied agents in this pharmacologic group [2]. Early studies of the drug using cystometrography in patients who had neurogenic bladders and upper motor neuron disorders proved the drug effective in controlling urinary urgency, frequency, and incontinence [3]. The US Food and Drug Administration (FDA) eventually approved oxybutynin in 1975 for the treatment of uninhibited and reflex neurogenic bladders and for the treatment of enuresis in patients older than 5 years.

In the early 1980s, oxybutynin was found efficacious not only for those who had neuropathic disturbances but also for patients who had detrusor overactivity without known neuropathic disturbance. In 1980, Moisey and colleagues [4] reported the results of a randomized double-blind study in 30 patients who had detrusor instability. Their findings suggested that the drug provided subjective improvement of symptoms in most of the patients treated, with urodynamic improvement in half of the patients completing the study. This study and others allowed oxybutynin to gain FDA approval for its use in detrusor instability in 1992. Over the last few decades, oxybutynin has demonstrated efficacy and safety in several clinical trials [5–7].

Not only has the evolution of oxybutynin expanded but its formulation has also been extended into a long-acting, controlled-release tablet. This formulation is available as a once-a-day dose and is FDA approved for overactive bladder. This formulation allowed practitioners great latitude in choosing the appropriate dose for the patient and allowing them to adjust the dose accordingly. Currently, physicians' options include immediate-release 5 mg, immediate-release 5 mg/5 mL syrup, and extended-release 5, 10, or 15 mg, with the ability to use as much as 30 mg daily.

* Corresponding author.
E-mail address: adiokno@beaumont.edu (A. Diokno).

Pharmacodynamics

Chemically, oxybutynin is *d,l* (racemic)-4-diethylamino-2-butynyl phenylcyclohexylglyconate, a tertiary amine (Fig. 1) [8]. Oxybutynin binds to parasympathetic muscarinic receptors with relative selectivity for M_3 and M_1 receptors compared with other subtypes, and may have higher affinity for parotid gland receptors than in the bladder. This relative selectivity may partially explain the relatively higher incidence of adverse side effects in conventional oxybutynin compared with other anticholinergics [9,10]. The anticholinergic properties of oxybutynin along with its antispasmodic activity are responsible for its relaxant effects on the detrusor muscle [8]. These properties allow increased bladder capacity, allow decreased frequency of uninhibited bladder contractions, and delay the initial desire to void [11]. In addition, oxybutynin resembles amines such as lidocaine and may have local anesthetic effects; however, the significance of this characteristic has been debated.

Pharmacokinetics

Following administration of oxybutynin chloride, plasma concentrations rise for 4 to 6 hours. The extended-release form allows steady plasma concentrations for up to 24 hours and minimizes the peak and trough concentrations seen with the conventional twice-daily dosage form (Fig. 2) [11,12]. Side effects of the conventional form were associated with peaks, whereas lower efficacy was related to troughs in concentration. Steady-state concentrations may be achieved after 72 hours of dosage of extended-release oxybutynin chloride. Hughes and colleagues [13] reported on the use of oxybutynin in the elderly population. Their findings showed a significant increase in maximum plasma concentration in "frail" elderly patients compared with healthy elderly control subjects, which may suggest that a lower dose

should be used for the aged population that has significant comorbidity. The wide spectrum of formulations of oxybutynin chloride and the dosing options available make oxybutynin an extremely easy and convenient drug to use in most patient populations.

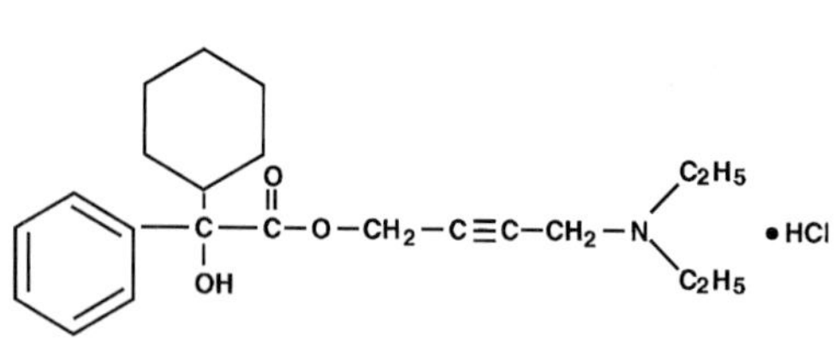

Metabolism

Oxybutynin chloride is rapidly absorbed by the gastrointestinal tract and metabolized primarily in the liver by the cytochrome P-450 CYP3A4 enzyme [11]. The extended-release form releases parent drug mainly in the lower gastrointestinal tract where cytochrome P-450 metabolism is less extensive. Metabolites of the drug include *N*-desethyl-oxybutynin, a biologically active metabolite, and phenylcyclohexylglycolic acid, which is inactive. Most adverse events related to the administration of conventional oxybutynin have been attributed to its active metabolite, and measurements of plasma levels of oxybutynin and *N*-desethyl-oxybutynin have shown a 5 to 11 fold higher area under the plasma concentration time curve for the metabolite [14]. Animal studies have shown that *N*-desethyl-oxybutynin binds significantly to muscarinic receptors in the bladder and the salivary glands, and receptor binding activity is similar to that of oxybutynin [15]. With the extended-release form, the metabolite formation is lower and the bioavailability of oxybutynin is higher than with the immediate-release form [16]. Others who have evaluated the drug's metabolism have shown no accumulation of oxybutynin or *N*-desethyl-oxybutynin during dosage with the controlled-release form [17].

Extended-release oxybutynin for detrusor overactivity

Four large clinical studies have evaluated the efficacy of extended-release oxybutynin in controlling one of the most common symptoms of overactive bladder, namely, urge urinary incontinence. Three of these four studies used patient-dependent, dose-adjustment strategies, which allowed physicians to balance efficacy with side effects. The remaining study was a forced dose-escalation study that compared extended-release oxybutynin to placebo. Patients reported an average of 16 to 28 weekly incontinence episodes before treatment. After treatment, extended-release oxybutynin consistently and dramatically

Fig. 1. Chemical makeup of oxybutynin. (*From* Oxybutynin chloride, package insert. Alza Corporation, Mountain View, California. June 2004; with permission.)

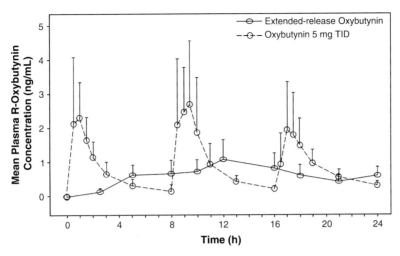

Fig. 2. Comparison of oxybutynin extended-release daily dosing to oxybutynin twice-daily dosing. (*From* Oxybutynin chloride, package insert. Alza Corporation, Mountain View, California. June 2004; with permission.)

reduced the mean number of weekly urge incontinence episodes. Patients reported a mean of 2 to 5 episodes a week post-treatment, corresponding to an 83% to 90% reduction in mean weekly incidents. Some patients (41%–50%) reported complete urinary continence, indicating that extended-release oxybutynin has the potential to eliminate the clinical manifestations of detrusor overactivity [18]. Information on other anticholinergic agents providing complete urinary continence is limited in the literature.

Comparison with other anticholinergics

The Overactive Bladder: Judging Effective Control and Treatment (OBJECT) trial was the first head-to-head study that compared extended-release oxybutynin with immediate-release tolterodine. This study took place at 37 centers and was a randomized, two-arm, parallel-group, double-blind, double-dummy trial that aimed to compare the efficacy and tolerability of 10 mg of daily extended-release oxybutynin with 2 mg of twice-daily immediate-release tolterodine. The secondary objective of this trial was to evaluate tolerability of both treatments—specifically, patient-reported adverse events. Extended-release oxybutynin reduced the number of weekly episodes of urge incontinence from 25.6 to 6.1, whereas tolterodine decreased the number of weekly episodes from 24.1 to 7.8. Extended-release oxybutynin demonstrated a statistically significant difference ($P = 0.03$) compared with tolterodine immediate-release. In addition,

patients receiving extended-release oxybutynin experienced significantly lower micturition frequency compared with tolterodine immediate-release ($P = 0.022$). Finally, extended-release oxybutynin showed a statistically significant difference in lowering the number of total or mixed incontinence episodes compared with tolterodine ($P = 0.022$). Adverse events were similar in each group, with no significant difference in the incidence of dry mouth, headache, constipation, or dyspepsia between the two groups [19].

With the advent of a long-acting preparation of tolterodine came the Overactive Bladder Performance of Extended-Release Agents (OPERA) trial. This trial was a randomized, double-blind, parallel-group study at multiple centers in the United States that sought to compare 10-mg extended-release oxybutynin with 4-mg long-acting tolterodine. A total of 790 patients, all women, were enrolled in the study. Patients had symptoms of 21 to 60 urge urinary incontinence episodes per week and 10 or more episodes of urgency and frequency in a 24-hour period. Patients taking extended-release oxybutynin had a 71% mean reduction in weekly urge incontinence and a 30% mean reduction in weekly micturition frequency, and 23% of patients achieved total dryness (Fig. 3). Although there was no statistically significant difference in the reduction of urge incontinence episodes and total incontinence episodes between the two study groups, there was a significant relative difference in reduction of micturition frequency of 13% ($P = 0.003$). Hence,

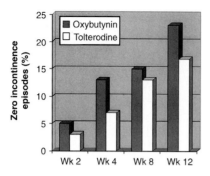

Fig. 3. Percentage of patients who had no episodes of urinary incontinence by study week (Wk). (*Adapted from* Diokno A, Appell R, Sand P, et al. OPERA Study Group. Prospective, randomized, double-blind study of the efficacy and tolerability of the extended-release formulations of oxybutynin and tolterodine for overactive bladder: results of the OPERA trial. Mayo Clin Proc 2003;78(6):691; with permission.)

this study concluded that 37% more patients achieved total dryness with extended-release oxybutynin compared with long-acting tolterodine ($P < 0.05$) [20].

Subanalysis of data from the OPERA trial was performed to evaluate the effects of controlled-release preparations of tolterodine and oxybutynin on nocturnal voiding frequency. Although both drugs provided a reduction of nocturnal voids compared with baseline, there was a significantly greater reduction of the number of nocturnal voiding episodes in younger patients (under 65 years) taking extended-release oxybutynin compared with those taking extended-release tolterodine. This finding suggests that controlled-release oxybutynin may be especially advantageous for young patients who find nocturnal voiding to be a bothersome symptom [21].

Evaluation of patients before treatment

In a prospective observational trial, 356 female patients who had reported symptoms of overactive bladder were evaluated with urodynamics before treatment with conventional oxybutynin chloride. Inclusion criteria were greater than seven voids per 24 hours and urgency with or without urge incontinence. Only 76% of these patients had urodynamic evidence of detrusor overactivity (defined as spontaneous, uninhibited increases in detrusor pressure during filling). All patients, regardless of urodynamic findings, were treated

with 2.5 mg of twice-daily oxybutynin chloride. Patients who had urodynamic detrusor overactivity and patients who did not have urodynamically verified symptoms had equal improvement in urinary frequency or incontinence episodes. Therefore, this study concluded that urodynamic testing is not necessary in patients who report symptoms of simple urgency, frequency, or urge urinary incontinence before starting treatment [22].

Safety and tolerability

The use of oxybutynin since the early 1960s has afforded clinicians the ability to thoroughly evaluate its safety and efficacy. One of the early clinical trials of oxybutynin evaluated it as therapy for irritable bowel syndrome and established its most common adverse events, namely, constipation, dry mouth, and visual disturbances. A secondary goal of the OBJECT trial was to evaluate tolerability of extended-release oxybutynin by patient-reported adverse events. In this study, most adverse events were those that would normally be expected in patients treated with anticholinergic agents. Dry mouth was reported in 28.1% of patients, with other side effects being headache (8.1%), constipation (7.0%), and dyspepsia (5.9%).

Extended-release oxybutynin was well tolerated in the OPERA study, with total dry mouth being the most common adverse event (29.7%), which was statistically different ($P < 0.05$) from those taking long-acting tolterodine (22.3%). Both groups showed a similar rate of discontinuation of therapy due to adverse events ($\sim 5\%$ for each group). Other adverse events noted in the study were mild or moderate dry mouth, diarrhea, constipation, headache, and urinary tract infection.

In a recent trial, extended-release oxybutynin was evaluated over up to a 12-month period to study the long-term safety profile. This multicenter trial followed a total of 904 women and 163 men using quality-of-life assessments to measure the impact of incontinence and evaluate treatment outcome with extended-release oxybutynin. In this study, most discontinuations were in the first 3 months (25.5%) and were related to adverse events, most commonly dry mouth (8.4%). Of those continuing after 3 months, 62% remained on extended-release oxybutynin for 1 year.

Patients had significant improvements in quality-of-life measures in this multicenter trial [23].

Because oxybutynin and its extended-release form are tertiary amines, they can theoretically cross the blood-brain barrier and produce central nervous system adverse events. Central nervous system adverse events of oxybutynin, including somnolence, dizziness, and insomnia, were limited in the OPERA study and were similar to tolterodine. The incidence of central nervous system adverse events was reported at rates between 1.2% and 4.3% for extended-release oxybutynin and between 1.1% and 5.2% for extended-release tolterodine over the entire study period. These adverse events led to early discontinuation by only 1.5% of the participants taking extended-release oxybutynin and 0.5% of participants taking extended-release tolterodine. This difference was not statistically significant [24].

Use in neurogenic bladder

Oxybutynin is widely used in patients who have neurogenic bladder dysfunction. Bennett and colleagues [25] evaluated the efficacy and safety of high-dose oxybutynin chloride in patients who had multiple sclerosis, spinal cord injury, and Parkinson's disease. This trial was a prospective, 12-week dose-titration trial of extended-release oxybutynin. Doses were increased by 5 mg at weekly intervals to a maximum dose of 30 mg daily. Patient perception of efficacy versus side effects directed dose escalation. Of 39 patients enrolled in the study, 22 had multiple sclerosis, 10 had spinal cord injury, and 7 had Parkinson's disease. Within 1 week of treatment, over half of the patients reported a decrease in the number of voids per day, and at the end of the study, there was a statistically significant decrease in 24-hour voids, episodes of nocturia, and incontinence episodes. Most (74.4%) patients in this study requested higher doses (15 mg or greater) of extended-release oxybutynin, and therefore, these investigators concluded that in this population, doses of up to 30 mg may be more effective [25].

Use in children

Oxybutynin has been used effectively for a number of years in the pediatric population. Early studies showed that conventional oxybutynin significantly increased bladder capacity and decreased intravesical pressure, leading to resolution or downgrading of vesicoureteral reflux [26]. Children who have uninhibited neurogenic bladder have benefited greatly from the use of the drug, with success rates of 90% [27]. Traditionally, conventional oxybutynin had to be dosed three times daily in children due to its pharmacokinetic properties. In adults who take oxybutynin, a steady drop in plasma concentration can be expected after 30 minutes of ingestion of the drug, whereas a more severe drop is seen in children [28].

More recently, Kogan and Youdim [29] evaluated the safety and efficacy of extended-release oxybutynin in children who had neurogenic bladder dysfunction and in children who had urinary urgency and frequency but not neurologic dysfunction. Dosage was as close to 0.3 mg/kg daily as possible using the available 5-, 10-, and 15-mg preparations available. All patients who had neurogenic bladder (n = 11) reported a reduction in the number of incontinence episodes between catheterizations. Of the children diagnosed with urgency, frequency, and urge incontinence (n = 11), all reported a cure in daytime incontinence with extended-release oxybutynin. Nearly half of the patients (48%) experienced no side effects. Of those who did, the most common side effects were dry mouth, constipation, heat intolerance, and drowsiness, occurring in 40%, 16%, 16%, and 12% of all patients, respectively. With the increasing use of extended-release oxybutynin in children, issues of compliance and tolerability can be greatly minimized.

Other routes of administration

Oxybutynin chloride has been reported to be effective when given intravesically, transdermally, or in intrarectal form. Saito and colleagues [30] reported their 3-year experience of using a modified intravesical form (oxybutynin chloride with hydroxypropylcellulose) in patients who had neurogenic overactive bladder and were not satisfied with the oral form of the drug or other therapies. Cystometrography was used to evaluate patients before treatment, at 1 week, and at 3 years after the initial intravesical treatment. This study was limited to six patients whose mean bladder capacity before treatment was 129.7 mL. Cystometrography studies revealed that bladder capacity increased to 283.5 mL and 286.8 mL at 1 week and 3 years post-treatment, respectively.

Transdermal forms of oxybutynin chloride are available and deliver the drug over a 3- to 4-day period after application to intact skin. Dmochowski and colleagues [31] evaluated transdermal oxybutynin and randomized 520 adult patients to receive 1.3, 2.6, or 3.9 mg daily. Voiding diaries and incontinence-specific quality of life were part of the evaluation. In this study, the highest dose (3.9 mg) was associated with a significant reduction in the number of weekly incontinence episodes and daily urinary frequency, significantly increased mean voided volume, and improved quality of life. Using 2.6 mg increased mean voided volume.

In a second large, randomized, double-blind trial, efficacy of 3.9-mg oxybutynin administered transdermally was compared with placebo. Oxybutynin significantly decreased the number of incontinent episodes per week compared with placebo ($P = 0.0165$). In addition, the transdermal form reduced micturition frequency and increased voided volumes. Side effects of the transdermal form were mainly related to the site of application. Dry mouth and other adverse events associated with the oral form and other anticholinergics were less common in transdermal oxybutynin [32].

Few studies have evaluated intrarectal administration of oxybutynin. In one Polish study, patients not tolerating oral oxybutynin were offered an intrarectal form of oxybutynin. Fifteen patients who consented to the study were given 5 mg of intrarectal oxybutynin chloride twice daily. After switching to the intrarectal route of administration, none of the patients chose to discontinue the treatment. All patients reported an improvement in their symptoms of overactivity, with 25% of patients claiming their symptoms had completely disappeared. Only 13.3% of patients reported mild-intensity dry mouth [33].

Although oxybutynin chloride has been studied in many routes of administration, the oral route is the most thoroughly evaluated and commonly used form. The enteral route of administration should be attempted first in most patients. Patients not tolerating oral oxybutynin can be tried on another form.

Summary

Oxybutynin is the most well-studied anticholinergic agent for detrusor overactivity, with research dating back to the 1960s when it was originally evaluated. Oxybutynin is extremely safe and effective in almost every population including children, the elderly, and those who have neurogenic bladder. With more preparations available and more dosing flexibility than any other anticholinergic medication on the market, oxybutynin remains the "gold standard" for first-line therapy for patients who have detrusor overactivity.

References

[1] Majewski R, Campbell K, Dykstra S, et al. Anticholinergic agents. Esters of 4-Dialkyl- (or 4-Polymethylene-) amino-2-butynols. J Med Chem 1965; 8(5):719–20.

[2] Wein A. Pharmacologic options for the overactive bladder. Urology 1998;51(2A):43–7.

[3] Diokno A, Lapides J. Oxybutynin: a new drug with analgesic and anticholinergic properties. J Urol 1972;108(2):307–9.

[4] Moisey C, Stephenson T, Brendler C. The urodynamic and subjective results of treatment of detrusor instability with oxybutynin chloride. Br J Urol 1980; 52(6):472–5.

[5] Gajewski J, Awad J. Oxybutynin versus propantheline in patients with multiple sclerosis and detrusor hyperreflexia. J Urol 1986;135(5):966–8.

[6] Hehir M, Fitzpatrick J. Oxybutynin and the prevention of urinary incontinence in spina bifida. Eur Urol 1985;11(4):254–6.

[7] Thuroff J, Bunke B, Ebner A, et al. Randomized, double-blind, multicenter trial on treatment of frequency, urgency and incontinence related to detrusor hyperactivity: oxybutynin versus propantheline versus placebo. J Urol 1991;145(4):831–6.

[8] Yarker YE, Goa KL, Fitton A. Oxybutynin. A review of its pharmacodynamic and pharmacokinetic properties, and its therapeutic use in detrusor instability. Drugs Aging 1995;6(3):243–62.

[9] Chapple C. Muscarinic receptor antagonists in the treatment of overactive bladder. Urology 2000; 55(Suppl 5A):33–46.

[10] Michel MA. Benefit-risk assessment of extended-release oxybutynin. Drug Saf 2005;25(12):867–76.

[11] Oxybutynin chloride, package insert. Alza Corporation, Mountain View, California. June 2004.

[12] Preik M, Albrecht D, O'Connell M, et al. Effect of controlled-release delivery on the pharmacokinetics of oxybutynin at different dosages: severity-dependent treatment of the overactive bladder. BJU Int 2004;94(6):821–7.

[13] Hughes KM, Lang JC, Lazare R, et al. Measurement of oxybutynin and its N-desethyl metabolite in plasma, and its application in pharmacokinetic studies in young, elderly and frail elderly volunteers. Xenobiotica 1992;22(7):859–69.

[14] Buyse G, Waldeck K, Verpoorten C, et al. Intravesical oxybutynin for neurogenic bladder dysfunction: less systematic side effects due to reduced first pass metabolism. J Urol 1998;160:892–6.

[15] Oki T, Kawashima A, Uchida M, et al. In vivo demonstration of muscarinic receptor binding activity of N-desethyl-oxybutynin, active metabolite of oxybutynin. Life Sci 2005;76(21):2445–56.

[16] Sathyan G, Chancellor M, Gupta S. Effect of OROS controlled-release delivery on the pharmacokinetics and pharmacodynamics of oxybutynin chloride. Br J Clin Pharmacol 2001;52:409–17.

[17] Nilsson C, Lukkari E, Haarala M, et al. Comparison of a 10-mg controlled release oxybutynin tablet with a 5-mg oxybutynin tablet in urge incontinent patients. Neurourol Urodyn 1997;16(6):533–42.

[18] Diokno A. The evolution of oxybutynin chloride. J Urol 2002;167(4) Suppl:182.

[19] Appell R, Sand P, Dmochowski R, et al. Prospective randomized controlled trial of extended-release oxybutynin chloride and tolterodine tartrate in the treatment of overactive bladder: results of the OBJECT Study. Mayo Clin Proc 2001;76:358–63.

[20] Diokno A, Appell R, Sand P, et al. OPERA Study Group. Prospective, randomized, double-blind study of the efficacy and tolerability of the extended-release formulations of oxybutynin and tolterodine for overactive bladder: results of the OPERA trial. Mayo Clin Proc 2003;78(6):687–95.

[21] Appell R, Boone T. Effects of extended-release formulations of oxybutynin and tolterodine on nocturnal voiding frequency on women with overactive bladder. Presented at the 35th Annual Meeting of the International Continence Society. Montreal, Canada, August 2005.

[22] Malone-Lee J, Henshaw D, Cummings K. Urodynamic verification of an overactive bladder is not a prerequisite for antimuscarinic treatment response. Br J Urol Int 2003;92(4):415–7.

[23] Diokno A, Sand P, Labasky R, et al. Long-term safety of extended-release oxybutynin chloride in a community-dwelling population of participants with overactive bladder: a one-year study. Int Urol Nephrol 2002;34(1):43–9.

[24] Chu F, Dmochowski R, Lama D, et al. Extended-release formulations of oxybutynin and tolterodine exhibit similar central nervous system tolerability profiles: a subanalysis of data from the OPERA trial. Am J Obstet Gynecol 2005;192(6):1849–54.

[25] Bennett N, O'Leary M, Patel A, et al. Can higher doses of oxybutynin improve efficacy in neurogenic bladder? J Urol 2004;171(2 Pt 1):749–51.

[26] Homsy Y, Nsouli I, Hamburger B, et al. Effects of oxybutynin on vesicoureteral reflux in children. J Urol 1985;134(6):1168–71.

[27] Kass E, Diokno A, Montealegre A. Enuresis—principles of management and result of treatment. J Urol 1979;121(6):794–6.

[28] Autret E, Jonville A, Dutertre J, et al. Plasma levels of oxybutynin chloride in children. Eur J Clin Pharmacol 1994;46(1):83–5.

[29] Kogan B, Youdim K. Preliminary study of the safety and efficacy of extended-release oxybutynin in children. Urology 2002;59:428–32.

[30] Saito M, Watanabe T, Tabuchi F, et al. Urodynamic effects and safety of modified intravesical oxybutynin chloride in patients with neurogenic detrusor overactivity: 3 years experience. Int J Urol 2004; 11(8):592–6.

[31] Dmochowski R, Sand P, Zinner N, et al. Comparative efficacy and safety of transdermal oxybutynin and oral tolterodine versus placebo in previously treated patients with urge and mixed urinary incontinence. Urology 2003;62(2):237–42.

[32] Bang L, Easthope S, Perry C. Transdermal oxybutynin: for overactive bladder. Drugs Aging 2003; 20(11):857–64.

[33] Radziszewski P, Borkowski A. [Therapeutic effects of intrarectal administration of oxybutynin]. Wiadomosci Lekarskie 2002;55(11–12):691–8 [Polish].

ELSEVIER
SAUNDERS

Urol Clin N Am 33 (2006) 447–453

UROLOGIC
CLINICS
of North America

Tolterodine for Treatment of Overactive Bladder

Jamie A. Kanofsky, MD, Victor W. Nitti, MD, FACS*

*Department of Urology, New York University School of Medicine, 150 East 32nd Street,
New York, NY 10016, USA*

Antimuscarinic agents have long been the primary pharmacologic treatment for the chronic and distressing syndrome of overactive bladder (OAB) [1,2]. Immediate-release (IR) oxybutynin was the most widely available agent throughout the world, but its use was limited by a high incidence of antimuscarinic side effects, most notably dry mouth, constipation, blurred vision, and cognitive impairment [3]. Such adverse events frequently resulted in poor patient compliance and discontinuation of treatment [3–5]. Subsequently, a need was identified for effective and better-tolerated agents that would improve compliance and persistence. From this need, tolterodine was developed as the first of this class of drugs specifically targeted for the treatment of OAB [6]. In vivo experiments in cats demonstrated greater muscarinic receptor affinity in the bladder versus the salivary glands [7,8]. In human studies, the "bladder-selective" profile for tolterodine proved to have less undesirable antimuscarinic side effects than oxybutynin, with similar efficacy [9–11]. As such, tolterodine has been associated with less dry mouth, gastrointestinal side effects, visual impairments, and cognitive deficits than oxybutynin IR [12,13].

Chemical structure and metabolism

Tolterodine is a tertiary amine with relatively low lipophilicity. It is a competitive muscarinic receptor antagonist without selectivity for any of the five muscarinic receptor subtypes (M_1–M_5). Tolterodine undergoes immediate and extensive first-pass hepatic metabolism, mainly by way of CYP 2D6–mediated oxidation and CYP 3A4–mediated N-dealkylation [14]. Its 5-hydroxymethyl metabolite (5-HM) is the product of the predominating CYP 2D6 pathway and is pharmacologically equipotent with tolterodine. In contrast, the other metabolites of tolterodine are not known to contribute to its therapeutic effect [15,16]. Individuals lacking the CYP 2D6 enzyme, known as "poor metabolizers," are not able to form the active metabolite 5-HM, and the pharmacologic effects are therefore mediated by unbound tolterodine alone [17]. In "extensive metabolizers," however, the sum of unbound tolterodine and 5-HM make up the pharmacologically active moiety [15,17]. Tolterodine is rapidly absorbed after oral administration of IR tablets, with the time to peak serum concentration (C_{max}) being 1 to 2 hours [15,18]. Food intake has no clinically relevant effect on the bioavailability of tolterodine [19].

Regarding the clearance and elimination of tolterodine, one study showed that 77% of radioactivity was recovered in the urine within 7 days after oral administration of ^{14}C-labeled tolterodine and 17% of radioactivity was recovered in the feces. Most of the administered dose, however, was excreted within 24 hours [18]. Tolterodine IR has a mean systemic clearance of 44 L/h and an elimination half-life of 1.9 to 3.6 hours in extensive metabolizers [15]. In these patients, 5-HM has an elimination half-life of 2.5 to 3.7 hours. In contrast, tolterodine clearance in poor metabolizers is five times lower (mean 9.0 L/h) and the elimination half-life is accordingly longer (7.5–11 hours) [15].

The extended-release (ER) formulation of tolterodine uses a drug delivery system that contains soluble microspheres [20]. The drug is slowly released as the outer layer of the microsphere dissolves, leading to consistent delivery of drug over a 24-hour period. This mechanism provides

---

* Corresponding author.
E-mail address: victor.nitti@nyumc.org (V.W. Nitti).

smooth serum concentrations of drug. Tolterodine exhibits linear pharmacokinetics, and pharmacokinetic equivalence has been demonstrated between once-daily 4-mg capsules of tolterodine ER and twice-daily 2-mg IR tablets [21]. In one study, serum drug levels were shown to fluctuate less with the ER formulation. In this study, steadier drug levels for the ER preparation were demonstrated by a median C_{max} that was only 75% of that observed with the IR formulation and by minimum serum concentration values that were 1.5 times higher. In addition, the time to maximum serum levels values and terminal half-lives for tolterodine and 5-HM were greater after administration of the ER formulation, which is consistent with a slower release of drug from the tolterodine ER capsules. Moreover, there is no effect on bioavailability when the ER formulation is taken with food [22].

Receptor affinity and organ selectivity

Although tolterodine has no selectivity for muscarinic receptor subtypes, it has been shown to have functional selectivity for the bladder over the salivary glands in the cat model [8,23]. As previously mentioned, 5-HM has a pharmacologic profile similar to the parent compound [23,24] and contributes significantly to the therapeutic effect of tolterodine [15,18]. Radioligand-binding studies have shown that tolterodine and 5-HM bind to human muscarinic receptors in vitro [23,24] and do not show selectivity between the five muscarinic receptor subtypes. In contrast, oxybutynin and darifenacin have 10 fold and 47 fold greater affinity, respectively, at muscarinic M_3 versus M_2 receptors [25]. Furthermore, tolterodine and 5-HM bind to muscarinic receptors with similar affinities in the guinea pig bladder and parotid gland, whereas oxybutynin and darifenacin show 6.5 fold and 46 fold selectivity, respectively, for parotid receptors compared with those in the bladder [25]. Similarly, in vivo studies have also shown that compared with oxybutynin, tolterodine and 5-HM show functional selectivity for the bladder over the salivary glands. Anesthetized cats were used to demonstrate that intravenous tolterodine and 5-HM produced more effective inhibition of acetylcholine-induced bladder contraction than of electrically evoked salivation [23,24]. The same studies demonstrated the opposite selectivity profile for oxybutynin: a twofold greater inhibitory effect on salivation than on bladder contraction.

Although tolterodine and oxybutynin are tertiary amines, tolterodine is 30 times less lipid-soluble than oxybutynin and crosses the blood-brain barrier to a lesser degree [13]. After administration of radiolabeled tolterodine to mice, the lowest tissue-to-blood radioactivity ratios were found in the brain, whereas the highest ratios were found in the organs of elimination [26]. These findings may explain the relatively low incidence of cognitive and central nervous system side effects [16,17]. Tolterodine has been shown to cause only minimal electroencephalographic changes, whereas oxybutynin has significant effects [13]. To date, this effect has not been proved to translate into a difference in cognitive function.

Tolterodine clinical experience with immediate-release formulation

Based on chemical structure, metabolism, and animal studies, tolterodine has many properties that should make it effective in the treatment of OAB, with less adverse events. More important, clinical trials and experience with tolterodine have shown its benefits, particularly with respect to the combined parameters of efficacy and tolerability ("clinical effectiveness"). The tolterodine clinical development program was the largest such program ever undertaken for a medication for the treatment of OAB [9]. At the time, eight phase III studies were conducted to evaluate the efficacy, safety, and tolerability of tolterodine in patients who had complaints of frequency, urgency, or urge incontinence. Four of these studies were conducted over a 4-week period, and four took place over a 12-week period. In 1997, Appell [9] reported on the pooled data of the four 12-week randomized, double-blind studies conducted in parallel at 134 centers in nine countries. Two of the studies compared 2-mg twice-daily tolterodine IR with 5-mg thrice-daily oxybutynin IR or placebo; one study compared 2-mg twice-daily tolterodine with 5-mg thrice-daily oxybutynin without placebo; and the last study compared two dosages of tolterodine (1 mg and 2 mg twice daily) with placebo. Eligible patients were of both sexes, were 18 years or older, and had an average of eight or more voids per 24 hours or an average of one or more episodes of incontinence per 24 hours. Efficacy measures included the number of voids per 24 hours, the number of incontinence episodes per 24 hours, and the mean urinary volume voided per micturition. The Patient

Perception of Bladder Condition (PPBC) scale was also used to evaluate efficacy. Adverse events, blood pressure measurements, and serum blood tests were used to evaluate safety and tolerability.

Of the 1120 patients enrolled in the four studies, 121 were randomized to 1-mg tolterodine, 474 to 2-mg tolterodine, 349 to oxybutynin, and 176 to placebo. More patients taking oxybutynin (27%) withdrew early from the study compared with patients taking 1-mg tolterodine (6%), 2-mg tolterodine (13%), or placebo (10%), which was found to be statistically significant ($P < 0.001$ for all). Seventy-five percent of the patients in these trials were female, and the mean age was 59 years. After 12 weeks of active treatment, the mean number of voids per 24 hours was decreased significantly from baseline (by approximately 20%) in both tolterodine groups and in the oxybutynin group. The pooled results also showed a significant decrease (40%–60%) in the number of incontinence episodes per 24 hours for both drugs compared with placebo ($P < 0.05$). Similarly, the pooled results showed a significant increase in volume voided per micturition for both drugs over placebo ($P < 0.001$). The mean volume voided increased by 18% to 28% from baseline measurements after taking either dose of tolterodine or oxybutynin for 12 weeks. Furthermore, the PPBC showed improvement after 12 weeks of treatment compared with baseline. The number of patients noting improvement was found to be significantly higher in the 2-mg tolterodine group ($P = 0.003$) and the 5-mg oxybutynin group ($P = 0.017$) than in the placebo group.

Ninety-three percent of the patients in the placebo group reported adverse effects compared with 74%, 75%, and 78% of patients treated with 1-mg tolterodine, 2-mg tolterodine, and placebo, respectively. The number of adverse events per patient was also higher in the oxybutynin group than in the other three groups. The most common side effect in all treatment groups was dry mouth, which was reported in 16% of the placebo group, 24% of the 1-mg tolterodine group, 40% of the 2-mg tolterodine group, and 78% of the oxybutynin group. The percentage of oxybutynin patients who had dry mouth was shown to be significantly higher compared with tolterodine or placebo patients ($P < 0.001$ for all comparisons), and the percentage of patients reporting moderate or severe dry mouth was also significantly higher in the oxybutynin group ($P < 0.001$ for all). Subsequently, the percentage of patients who discontinued the study due to adverse events

was significantly higher in the oxybutynin group than in the tolterodine groups or the placebo group ($P < 0.001$ for all). Serious adverse events were evenly distributed throughout the groups. Specifically, 3% of patients in the placebo group, 4% in each tolterodine group, and 4% in the oxybutynin group experienced serious events. Furthermore, blood pressure and laboratory values indicated no significant differences between the treatment groups, reinforcing the notion that tolterodine is as safe as oxybutynin and placebo.

By pooling the results of the four phase III clinical trials involving more than 1100 patients, Appell [9] was able to document that tolterodine IR was as efficacious as oxybutynin and had a greater tolerability profile at equivalent doses. Not only did the tolterodine patients experience significantly fewer occurrences of dry mouth, overall adverse events, and study withdrawals, but 70% continued taking tolterodine for greater than 12 months, with reported maintenance of efficacy. These data served as the stepping stone for further advancements in the management of patients who have OAB.

Tolterodine extended-release formulation

Although multiple large, multicenter studies and initial clinical experience confirmed the efficacy and tolerability of tolterodine IR for OAB, it requires twice-daily administration. Subsequently, an ER formulation was developed to provide a sustained release of the drug over a 24-hour period. An ER formulation provides a more convenient once-daily dosage and certain metabolic advantages. Tolterodine ER has a flatter serum concentration-time profile compared with the IR formulation, thus minimizing peak and trough levels. In 2001, Van Kerrebroeck and colleagues [6] reported the first large, multicenter, placebo-controlled study of tolterodine ER designed to evaluate its efficacy and tolerability and to determine whether the ER formulation provided additional improvements in efficacy and tolerability relative to the IR formulation.

This randomized, double-blind, placebo-controlled study was conducted in 167 centers in Australia, Asia, Europe, and North America. A total of 1529 women and men were randomized to 4-mg once-daily tolterodine ER, 2-mg twice-daily tolterodine IR, or placebo for 12 weeks. Treatment efficacy was assessed by comparing the changes in the urinary diary variables from baseline to week 12. Tolterodine ER ($P = 0.0001$) and tolterodine IR ($P = 0.0005$) showed statistically significant reductions in the number of incontinence episodes compared with placebo. In addition, the ER formulation was 18% more effective in reducing incontinence episodes than the IR formulation ($P < 0.05$). Furthermore, the mean total micturition frequency for patients taking the ER formulation decreased by 25% from baseline, demonstrating a 59% improvement over placebo ($P = 0.0001$). Tolerability was also improved with the ER formulation. Among all three treatment groups, the most common adverse events were dry mouth, constipation, and headache. All side effects other than dry mouth were seen in equal distribution in the treatment and placebo groups. The incidence of dry mouth in the IR group was 30%, whereas it was 23% ($P < 0.02$) in the ER group. Only 1.8% of patients taking the ER formulation complained of severe dry mouth. Thus, the ER formulation showed significant advantages over the IR formulation, with a decrease in the number of incontinence episodes and a lower incidence of dry mouth.

Tolterodine comparator trials

The first comparator trial using tolterodine was the Overactive Bladder: Judging Effective Control and Treatment (OBJECT) study. This study sought to evaluate the efficacy and tolerability of oxybutynin ER versus tolterodine IR after 12 weeks of treatment [27]. This randomized, double-blind, parallel-group study done at 37 United States sites was conducted in a fairly severe OAB population. Patients who had 7 to 50 episodes of urge incontinence per week and 10 or more voids in a 24-hour period were randomized to receive 10-mg once-daily oxybutynin ER or 2-mg twice-daily tolterodine IR. A total of 378 patients of both sexes (315 women and 63 men) were randomized to the two treatment arms. At the end of the 12-week study period, both drugs were shown to improve symptoms of OAB significantly from baseline as evaluated by the three main outcome measures. Specifically, 96.2% and 95.3% of the patients using oxybutynin ER and tolterodine IR, respectively, had less episodes of incontinence at the end of the study. The investigators, however, found the ER formulation of oxybutynin to be slightly more effective than tolterodine IR in each of the main outcome measures adjusted for baseline—number of

episodes of urge incontinence ($P = 0.4$), total incontinence ($P = 0.03$), and micturition frequency ($P = 0.02$). Tolerability (specifically, dry mouth) was similar in both groups (28.1% for oxybutynin ER and 33.2% for tolterodine IR).

The follow-up study to the OBJECT study was the Overactive Bladder: Performance of Extended Release Agents (OPERA) study that compared the efficacy and tolerability of ER formulations of tolterodine (4 mg daily) and oxybutynin (10 mg daily) [28]. This randomized, double-blind, active-control study enrolled 790 women at 71 United States study centers. OPERA used similar outcome parameters: final weekly episodes of urge incontinence (primary outcome measure), final weekly total incontinence episodes, and weekly micturition frequency. There was no statistical difference found between the average weekly urge urinary incontinence episodes or total dryness in the oxybutynin ER group and the tolterodine ER group. Twenty-three percent of the oxybutynin participants reported total dryness and 26.7% denied urge urinary incontinence episodes in their week-12 voiding diary, whereas only 16.8% of tolterodine participants reported total dryness and 20.9% reported lack of any urge urinary incontinence episodes at last assessment. Patients on oxybutynin had a slightly lower weekly micturition frequency at the end of the 12-week study ($P = 0.003$). The most common side effect in each group was dry mouth, with 29.7% of the patients receiving oxybutynin reporting dry mouth compared with 22.3% of the tolterodine patients ($P = 0.02$). Other adverse events were similar in magnitude and frequency for both groups. More importantly, neither drug used in the study caused any serious adverse events. The OPERA study did have a few limitations: the participants were solely women who had a large number of urge urinary incontinence episodes per week (21–60), which may be somewhat atypical of the general OAB population.

The Antimuscarinic Clinical Effectiveness Trial (ACET) assessed a diverse "real-world" population of patients who had OAB [29]. A global measure of efficacy (the PPBC) was used as the primary end point [30]. In addition, dry mouth was assessed with a visual analog scale (VAS). Approximately one half of the patients received the higher dose and one half received the lower dose in each study arm. This study involved the use of open-label medications in two separate trials: one with patients randomized to 2 mg or 4 mg of tolterodine ER and the other with patients randomized to 5 mg or 10 mg of oxybutynin ER. The trials were conducted in parallel at 340 centers in the United States, and each center evaluated only one of the drugs being studied. The trial recruited patients of both sexes 18 years or older who had OAB. After enrolling, patients were randomized to treatment with one of the two doses (2 mg versus 4 mg for tolterodine subjects or 5 mg versus 10 mg for oxybutynin patients) to be taken once daily for an 8-week period. A total of 1289 patients were enrolled in the study: 620 in the oxybutynin trial and 669 in the tolterodine trial. Seventy percent of the patients taking 4-mg tolterodine ER, 60% of those taking 2-mg tolterodine ER, 59% of the 5-mg oxybutynin ER patients, and 60% of the 10-mg oxybutynin ER patients perceived at least a 1-point improvement in their bladder condition on the PPBC scale after taking the medication for 8 weeks. The greater-perceived improvement attributed to 4-mg tolterodine ER over 10-mg oxybutynin ER was found to be statistically significant ($P < 0.01$) in both cases. The primary reason for early discontinuation of the study was adverse events. A significantly greater percentage of patients in the 10-mg oxybutynin group than in the 4-mg tolterodine group withdrew due to side effects (13% versus 6%, $P = 0.001$). Using a VAS, patients taking the higher doses of both medications (tolterodine and oxybutynin) complained of more severe dry mouth than their counterparts taking the lower dosages. Patients taking 4-mg tolterodine ER, however, reported a significantly lower severity of dry mouth than those taking 10-mg oxybutynin ER ($P = 0.03$).

The ACET study efficacy end points were based solely on a subjective global parameter (PPBC), and the side effect end point was a VAS, neither of which had been used previously in OAB medication trials. Indeed, these variables add a novel aspect to the study, but the results must be interpreted with caution. Other limitations include the open-label nature of the study, which may create patient and physician bias, and the short 8-week time frame of the study.

The most recent comparator trial of tolterodine tested the efficacy and tolerability of tolterodine versus the newer antimuscarinic, solifenacin [31]. The STAR trial (Solifenacin and Tolterodine as an Active Comparator in a Randomized trial) was a prospective, double-blind, double-dummy, parallel-group study that was conducted over a 12-week time period [31]. This trial was powered to show noninferiority of solifenicin in the primary efficacy variable of change in number of micturitions per 24 hours. In addition, a number of secondary efficacy variables were measured. These included episodes of urgency, urge incontinence, incontinence (with and without the sensation of urgency), and nocturia, the proportion of patients who experienced a 50% reduction in incontinence episodes, and the number of patients who were incontinent at baseline but continent at study end point.

This trial was unique in that it used the recommended doses of both compounds in a manner consistent with product labeling while allowing patients the option to increase their dose (only available for solifenacin) depending on satisfaction with treatment efficacy and tolerability. Initially, patients were entered into a 2-week single-blind placebo run-in whereby they completed a 3-day voiding diary before randomization. Eligibility criteria included an average of eight or greater micturitions per 24 hours, an average of one or more episodes of incontinence per 24 hours, or an average of one or more episodes of urgency per 24 hours. After enrolling, patients were randomized to 5-mg daily solifenacin or to 4-mg daily tolterodine ER. The patients then had the option to continue the initial drug dose or to increase the dosage after 4 weeks of treatment. However, because tolterodine is not approved in dosages greater than 4 mg/d, the patients randomized to this group who chose the dose increase continued taking the 4-mg dose plus placebo.

The primary efficacy outcome showed that treatment with solifenacin was "noninferior" to tolterodine ER with regard to the change from baseline in mean number of micturitions per 24 hours (-2.45 for solifenicin versus -2.24 for tolterodine). Solifenacin showed statistically significant improvements from baseline in urgency ($P = 0.035$), urge incontinence ($P = 0.001$), and overall incontinence ($P = 0.006$) over tolterodine. It is of interest that 51% of the patients treated with tolterodine ER and 48% of those treated with solifenacin requested an increase in dosage after 4 weeks of treatment due to inadequate therapeutic benefit on the initial dose.

Although the STAR trial claimed improved efficacy of solifenacin over tolterodine, the results must be interpreted carefully. The trial was designed as a "noninferiority study," and it was just that. One must carefully draw conclusions based on secondary efficacy variables for a study powered to the primary efficacy variable. In addition, due to the study design, patients were allowed to request an increase in medication dosage at the 4-week mark if not optimally satisfied with their initial therapeutic results. The patients randomized to tolterodine ER, however, were kept at their initial 4-mg daily dosage (keeping in line with recommended dosage use), whereas those receiving solifenacin were increased from 5 to 10 mg daily (allowing those seeking a higher dose to get it). With a doubling of medication dosage in one group, it is expected that the efficacy results would improve accordingly. Of note, a substantial increase in adverse effects accompanied the improved efficacy. It can certainly be argued that this trial represents a more realistic clinical use of the drugs according to regulatory standards; however, as expected, the improvement in efficacy is accompanied by an increase in side effects. This study demonstrated that multidose solifenacin may have a slightly better efficacy profile, whereas tolterodine ER possesses a more desirable tolerability profile.

Summary

Tolterodine was developed in response to the need for a more bladder-specific antimuscarinic agent with fewer side effects. For patients who have OAB, this drug's functional selectivity seen in animal models has translated into similar efficacy and improved tolerability over its predecessors. Comparator studies have shown tolterodine to be equal in efficacy to other agents while possessing a favorable side effect profile, especially with respect to dry mouth. Tolterodine was developed specifically with tolerability in mind. It was never registered at higher doses that might offer better efficacy in patients requiring greater antimuscarinic doses. The IR and the ER formulations of tolterodine remain an important option for the treatment of OAB.

References

[1] Andersson K-E. The overactive bladder: pharmacologic basis of drug treatment. Urology 1997; 50(Suppl 6A):74–84.

[2] Abrams P, Larsson G, Chapple C, et al. Factors involved in the success of antimuscarinic treatment. BJU Int 1999;83(Suppl 2):42–7.

[3] Yarker Y, Goa KL, Fitton A. Oxybutynin: a review of its pharmacodynamic and pharmacokinetic properties, and its therapeutic use in detrusor instability. Drugs Aging 1995;6:243–62.

[4] Thuroff J, Bunke B, Ebner A, et al. Randomized, double-blind multicenter trial on treatment of

frequency, urgency, and incontinence related to detrusor hyperactivity: oxybutynin versus propantheline versus placebo. J Urol 1991;145:813–7.

[5] Appell RA, Abrams P, Drutz HP, et al. Treatment of overactive bladder: long-term tolerability and efficacy of tolterodine. World J Urol 2001;19:141–7.

[6] Van Kerrebroeck P, Kreder K, Jonas U, et al. Tolterodine once-daily: superior efficacy and tolerability in the treatment of the overactive bladder. Urology 2001;57:414–21.

[7] Nilvebrant L. The mechanism of action of tolterodine. Rev Contemp Pharmacother 2000;11:13–27.

[8] Stahl MMS, Eckstrom B, Sparf A, et al. Urodynamic and other effects of tolterodine: a novel antimuscarinic drug for the treatment of detrusor overactivity. Neurourol Urodyn 1995;14:647–55.

[9] Appell R. Clinical efficacy and safety of tolterodine in the treatment of overactive bladder: a pooled analysis. Urology 1997;50(Suppl 6A):90–6.

[10] Abrams P, Freeman R, Anderstrom C, et al. Tolterodine, a new antimuscarinic agent: as effective but better tolerated than oxybutynin in patients with an overactive bladder. Br J Urol 1998;81(6):801–10.

[11] Drutz HP, Appell RA, Gleason D, et al. Clinical efficacy and safety of tolterodine compared to oxybutynin and placebo in patients with overactive bladder. Int Urogyn J 1999;10(5):283–9.

[12] Chapple CR, Nilvebrant L. Tolterodine: selectivity for the urinary bladder over the eye (as measured by visual accommodation) in healthy volunteers. Drugs R D 2002;3(2):75–81.

[13] Todorova A, Vonderheid-Guth B, Dimpfel W. Effects of tolterodine, trospium chloride, and oxybutynin on the central nervous system. J Clin Pharmacol 2001;41:636–44.

[14] Postlind H, Danielson A, Lindgren A, et al. Tolterodine, a novel muscarinic receptor antagonist, is metabolized by cytochromes P450 2D6 and 3A in human liver microsomes. Drug Metab Dispos 1998;26(4):289–93.

[15] Brynne N, Dalen P, Alvan G, et al. Influence of CYP2D6 polymorphism on the pharmacokinetics and pharmacodynamics of tolterodine. Clin Pharmacol Ther 1998;63(5):529–39.

[16] Hills CJ, Winter SA, Balfour JA. Tolterodine. Drugs 1998;55:813–20.

[17] Clemett D, Jarvis B. Tolterodine: a review of its use in the treatment of overactive bladder. Drugs Aging 2001;18(4):277–304.

[18] Brynne N, Stahl MMS, Hallen B, et al. Pharmacokinetics and pharmacodynamics of tolterodine in man: a new drug for the treatment of urinary bladder overactivity. Int J Clin Pharmacol Ther 1997;35: 287–95.

[19] Olsson B, Brynne N, Johansson C. Food increases the bioavailability of tolterodine but not effective exposure. J Clin Pharmacol 2001;41(3):298–304.

[20] Rovner ES, Wein AJ. Once-daily, extended-release formulations of antimuscarinic agents in the

treatment of overactive bladder: a review. Eur Urol 2002;41:6–14.

[21] Olsson B, Szamosi J. Multiple-dose pharmacokinetics of a new once-daily, extended-release tolterodine formulation versus immediate-release tolterodine. Clin Pharmacokinet 2001;40(3):227–35.

[22] Olsson B, Szamosi J. Food does not influence the pharmacokinetics of a new, extended-release formulation of tolterodine for once daily treatment of patients with overactive bladder. Clin Pharmacokinet 2001;40(2):135–43.

[23] Nilvebrant L, Andersson K-E, Gillberg P-G, et al. Tolterodine—a new bladder-selective antimuscarinic agent. Eur J Pharm 1997;327:195–207.

[24] Nilvebrant L, Hallen B, Larsson G. Tolterodine: a new bladder selective, muscarinic receptor antagonist: pre-clinical pharmacological and clinical data. Life Sci 1997;60:1129–36.

[25] Nilvebrant L, Gillberg P-G, Sparf B. Antimuscarinic potency and bladder selectivity of PNU-200577, a major metabolite of tolterodine. Pharmacol Toxicol 1997;81:169–72.

[26] Nilvebrant L, Pahlman I, d'Argy R. Tissue distribution of tolterodine and its metabolites: low penetration into the central nervous system. Presented at the 15th Meeting of the European Association of Urology. Brussels, April 12–15, 2000.

[27] Appell RA, Sand PK, Dmochowski RR, et al. Prospective randomized controlled trial of extended-release oxybutynin chloride and tolterodine tartrate in the treatment of overactive bladder: results of the OBJECT study. Mayo Clin Proc 2001;76:358–63.

[28] Diokno AC, Appell RA, Sand PK, et al. Prospective, randomized, double-blind study of the efficacy and tolerability of the extended-release formulations of oxybutynin and tolterodine for overactive bladder: results of the OPERA trial. Mayo Clin Proc 2003; 78:687–95.

[29] Sussman D, Garely A. Treatment of overactive bladder with once-daily extended-release tolterodine or oxybutynin: the Antimuscarinic Clinical Effectiveness Trial (ACET). Cur Med Res Opin 2002;18: 177–84.

[30] Coyne KS, Matza LS, Kopp Z, et al. The validation of the Patient Perception of Bladder Condition (PPBC): a single-item global measure for patients with overactive bladder. Eur Urol 2006 Jan 24 [Epub ahead of print].

[31] Chapple CR, Martinez-Garcia R, Selvaggi L, et al. A comparison of the efficacy and tolerability of solifenacin succinate and extended release tolterodine at treating overactive bladder syndrome: results of the STAR trial. Eur Urol 2005;48:464–70.

ELSEVIER
SAUNDERS

Urol Clin N Am 33 (2006) 455–463

UROLOGIC
CLINICS
of North America

Transdermal Oxybutynin for Overactive Bladder

G. Willy Davila, MD[a],*, Jonathan S. Starkman, MD[b], Roger R. Dmochowski, MD[b]

[a]*Department of Gynecology, Section of Urogynecology and Reconstructive Pelvic Surgery, Cleveland Clinic Florida, 2950 Cleveland Clinic Boulevard, Weston, FL 33331, USA*
[b]*Department of Urologic Surgery, Vanderbilt University Medical Center, A-1302 Medical Center North, Nashville, TN 37232-2765, USA*

Overactive bladder is commonly treated with oral anticholinergic drugs such as oxybutynin chloride. Although oral anticholinergic agents have been effective in controlling urinary urgency and frequency and in decreasing incontinence episodes, adverse events, particularly dry mouth, often cause patients to discontinue oral therapy and to endure incontinence. Oxybutynin can be delivered transcutaneously, maintaining the efficacy of oral oxybutynin while significantly minimizing the side effects (eg, dry mouth) that may complicate therapy. By avoiding hepatic and gastrointestinal metabolism of oxybutynin, less N-desethyloxybutynin is produced (this compound is deemed responsible for the anticholinergic side effects such as dry mouth). This novel oxybutynin formulation offers patients who have overactive bladder and urge urinary incontinence a well-tolerated option for managing the symptoms of overactive bladder.

Pharmacotherapy for overactive bladder (OAB) primarily consists of oral anticholinergic medications. Antimuscarinic properties of these drugs block acetylcholine-induced stimulation of the postganglionic parasympathetic muscarinic receptor sites in animal [1,2] and human tissues [3]. A variety of pharmacologic agents are currently used for OAB. These agents are described elsewhere in this issue of the *Urologic Clinics of North America* and have been demonstrated to be effective in the treatment of OAB. Their effectiveness, however, is limited by their anticholinergic side effects and based primarily on their effect on muscarinic receptors outside of the bladder. More than one muscarinic receptor subtype can exist within a tissue or cell [4]. As such, both M_2 and M_3 receptors are present in the bladder. M_2 receptors account for 80% of the receptor concentration in the bladder and are responsible for detrusor relaxation. Conversely, M_3 receptors control detrusor contraction. About 90% of the muscarinic receptors in the salivary glands are of the M_3 variety [5]. It is the concomitant stimulation of these receptors by anticholinergic agents that leads to the well-recognized adverse side effects of dry mouth and constipation.

Oxybutynin pharmacologic effects on the bladder

Oxybutynin (OXY) has been used for decades to control the symptoms of urge urinary incontinence (UI). With spasmolytic and antimuscarinic properties, OXY has a direct relaxant effect on the bladder [6].

Oxy has been characterized as a muscarinic M_1/M_3 selective antagonist [7] and has a tenfold higher affinity for M_3 receptors than for M_2 receptors [4]. Therefore, this agent acts directly on the primary receptor responsible for detrusor contraction, explaining the drug's effectiveness in reducing urge UI episodes. It also acts on the primary receptors located in the salivary gland, explaining the associated incidence of dry mouth (87%) experienced by patients who take oral OXY [8].

Oral OXY formulations undergo extensive hepatic and gastrointestinal presystemic

---

* Corresponding author.
E-mail address: davilag@ccf.org (G.W. Davila).

metabolism to form a primary active metabolite, N-desethyloxybutynin (N-DEO). Following oral administration of the immediate-release OXY, N-DEO is present in the circulation at levels 4 to 10 times higher than that of the parent compound.

Oral OXY is very effective in reducing the number of weekly UI episodes, as demonstrated in multiple controlled trials. Although effectiveness is high, so is the incidence of dry mouth— 87% for extended-release OXY and 68% for immediate-release OXY [8]. Investigations into other OXY formulations and drug delivery systems were expanded, with the aim of reducing the incidence of anticholinergic side effects while maintaining the beneficial effects on OAB.

Rationale for transdermal drug delivery systems

Commercially available since the early 1980s, transdermal drug delivery systems (patches) continuously deliver drug molecules through the skin into the circulation. These systems maintain constant drug plasma levels and may simplify drug administration. The first transdermal drug delivery systems were patches that released the anti–motion sickness drug scopolamine. Nitroglycerin patches for angina prophylaxis soon followed, and today, a wide array of drugs are effectively administered by transdermal delivery.

Transdermal drug patches are available in two basic designs: one that controls the rate of drug delivery to the skin (reservoir type) and another that uses the skin to control the absorption rate (matrix type). Transdermal drug patches provide patients with ease of administration, disposability, and control of drug delivery. An added benefit is that first-pass metabolism by the liver can be avoided, permitting reduced drug doses and a reduction in drug interactions. The serum level peaks and troughs that are observed with immediate-release or even with extended-release oral medications are far less frequent with transdermal administration. Fewer side effects may promote patient compliance and increased treatment efficacy.

Transdermal oxybutynin

Based on its metabolism and side effect profile following oral administration, rationale exists for the use of transdermal OXY (TD-OXY). Following oral administration, agents undergo gastrointestinal and hepatic first-pass metabolism that can

reduce bioavailability [9,10]. Transdermal delivery systems allow the drug to bypass the gastrointestinal and hepatic first-pass metabolism, providing for more consistent control of absorption into the circulation [11]. Following oral administration, inconsistent serum drug concentrations may lead to adverse effects during unnecessarily high peak concentrations and subtherapeutic levels at trough times [9]. During transdermal therapy, more controlled absorption results in the ability to administer lower dosages and achieve therapeutic blood levels at a steady state over extended periods of time [12,13]. These lower dosages can lead to a reduction in dose-related side effects and ultimately lead to improved patient adherence. Because of its metabolite-related adverse effects, OXY is a prime candidate for transdermal delivery.

Chemistry

TD-OXY delivers the compound as the free base (not as a hydrochloride salt, as does the oral formulation). OXY is soluble in alcohol but relatively insoluble in water [14].

System characteristics

Approved by the US Food and Drug Administration in February 2003, TD-OXY is marketed as a matrix-type system composed of three layers (Fig. 1) [14]. The first layer consists of a thin backing film made of flexible and occlusive polyester/ethylene-vinyl acetate that ensures physical integrity and protects the middle layer, which contains the acrylic adhesive. This middle layer also contains OXY, triacetin, and United States Pharmacopeia, a plasticizer. The third layer is a release liner composed of two overlapping siliconized polyester strips that can be peeled off and

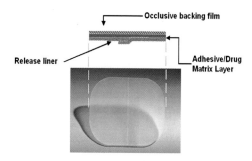

Fig. 1. Side and top views of the TD-OXY matrix system. (*Adapted from* Oxytrol package insert. Corona (CA): Watson Pharma, Inc.; 2003.)

discarded by the patient before applying the adhesive/drug layer to the skin.

Pharmacokinetics and metabolism

Absorption

The average daily dose of OXY absorbed from the 39-cm^2 patch is 3.9 mg. In a study of healthy volunteers, the average plasma OXY concentration during a single application of the 39-cm^2 system was 3 to 4 ng/mL in 24 to 48 hours, with steady concentrations maintained up to 96 hours (Fig. 2). This sustained delivery makes it possible for patients to apply a single patch for 3 to 4 days with effective round-the-clock maintenance of serum levels.

Like the oral formulation, TD-OXY is metabolized primarily by the cytochrome P-450 enzymes (particularly CYP3A4) found mostly in the liver and gut wall. Its metabolites include phenylcyclohexylglycolic acid, which is pharmacologically inactive, and N-DEO, which is pharmacologically active. Following oral administration of OXY, presystemic first-pass metabolism results in bioavailability of approximately 6% and a relatively higher plasma concentration of the active N-DEO

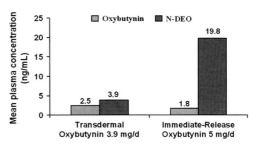

Fig. 3. Average plasma OXY and N-DEO concentrations measured up to 96 hours after transdermal or oral (extended-release) oxybutynin delivery.

metabolite compared with that following transdermal delivery [11,15]. Transdermal administration of OXY bypasses the gastrointestinal and hepatic first-pass metabolism, reducing the formation of N-DEO, even when compared with extended-release OXY (Fig. 3).

Pharmacokinetics

A pharmacokinetic study comparing transdermal with extended-release OXY demonstrated that transdermal administration resulted in considerably lower fluctuation in OXY and N-DEO plasma concentrations, reduced N-DEO formation, and increased saliva production during the dosing period [16]. Compared with oral administration, TD-OXY is administered at lower dosages yet is absorbed at higher levels; approximately 100% of the 3.9 mg is absorbed through the skin and into the circulation.

Adhesion

Because the pharmacologic agent is located in the adhesive layer, patch adhesion is critical to drug dosing. Adhesion was periodically evaluated during the phase III studies [9,17]. Of the 4746 evaluations of the transdermal system in these studies, 20 (0.4%) patches were observed at clinic visits to be completely detached and 35 (0.7%) were partially detached during routine clinical use. Therefore, more than 98% of the systems were assessed as at least 75% attached and would be expected to deliver adequate amounts of medication.

Clinical efficacy

One phase II study and two phase III studies were undertaken and demonstrated that TD-OXY is effective in controlling OAB symptoms, with

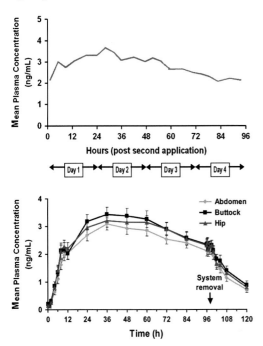

Fig. 2. Steady-state OXY concentrations following a single transdermal system application (top) on lower abdomen and (bottom) at different body sites. (*Data from* Oxytrol package insert. Corona (CA): Watson Pharma, Inc.; 2003.)

subsequent low incidence of anticholinergic side effects.

Phase II study

The phase II study was designed to maximize OXY dosage based on tolerability of dry mouth rather than on efficacy in reducing OAB symptoms. It was a double-blind, placebo-controlled trial of 249 urge UI patients who were currently responding to immediate-release OXY [9]. Symptom requirements recorded in a 3-day urinary diary after prestudy treatment washout included 10 or more urge UI episodes, 56 or more voids, and 350 mL or less urinary void volume. The efficacy end points included change from baseline in the number of incontinence episodes, comparisons of daily urinary frequency, and urinary voided volume. Safety end points were confirmation of continued efficacy and adherence. Double-blind therapy included twice-weekly application of TD-OXY, daily ingestion of oral OXY capsules, or matching placebo for 2 weeks. The dosage was then increased if the subject tolerated the dry-mouth symptomatology. The maximum oral dosage was 20 mg/d and the transdermal dosage was 5.2 mg/d. This phase II study was a short-term, 6-week study.

Results of the study showed that daily incontinence episodes decreased similarly in the transdermal and in the oral treatment groups (7.3 to 2.4 [66%] and 7.4 to 2.6 [72%], respectively, $P = 0.39$) [9]. The visual analog scale reduction in urinary leakage improved from washout in both groups ($P < 0.0001$), with no difference between them ($P = 0.9$). Most important, dry mouth occurred in significantly fewer patients in the transdermal group (38%) compared with the oral group (94%, $P < 0.001$) at the maximal achieved dosage. An anticholinergic symptoms questionnaire was used to capture the symptom of dry mouth unequivocally. Among patients in the transdermal group, 67% experienced a reduction in severity of dry mouth compared with previous oral treatment; 90% had no or mild skin erythema. Plasma concentrations of OXY increased according to dose and reflected differences in metabolism of transdermal versus oral administration, with N-DEO levels relatively low in the transdermal group. Overall, TD-OXY efficacy was comparable to that of oral immediate-release OXY, with a markedly lower incidence of dry mouth, giving credence to the concept of administration of OXY by way of transdermal routes.

Phase III studies

The first phase III study was a double-blind, placebo-controlled trial with 520 urge and mixed UI patients, with the goal of identifying the optimal dosage of TD-OXY [17]. Of the 520 patients, 125 received TD-OXY, 3.9 mg/d; 130 received TD-OXY, 1.3 mg/d; 133 received TD-OXY, 2.6 mg/d; and 132 received a placebo patch. After a 3- to 4-week screening period, patients continued treatment for 12 weeks. Symptom requirements recorded in a 7-day urinary diary after the prestudy washout period included 10 or more urge UI episodes and 56 or more voids. Efficacy end points of the study were the change from baseline in the number of incontinence episodes, daily urinary frequency comparisons, and urinary voided volume. Safety end points were the confirmation of continued efficacy and patient compliance.

In the study, the 3.9-mg daily dose of TD-OXY significantly decreased the number of weekly incontinence episodes (median change, -19.0 versus -15.0; $P = 0.0265$), reduced the average daily urinary frequency (median change, -2.0 versus -1.0; $P = 0.0313$), increased the average voided volume (median change, 26 mL versus 5.5 mL; $P = 0.0009$), and significantly improved quality of life (Incontinence Impact Questionnaire total score; $P = 0.0327$) compared with placebo. The most common adverse event was application-site pruritus (TD-OXY, 16.8%; placebo, 6.1%). The incidence of dry mouth in the transdermal group was similar to placebo (9.6% versus 8.3%). In the 12-week open-label period, a sustained reduction of nearly three incontinence episodes per day was noted for both groups.

The second phase III study compared the efficacy and safety of TD-OXY (3.9 mg/d) with oral, extended-release tolterodine (4 mg/d) and with placebo in 361 patients who had urge or mixed UI [18]. To study a more homogeneous population and to reduce side effect occurrence, all enrolled subjects were anticholinergic non-naïve, having been on previous pharmacotherapy for their OAB. Patients were randomized to 12 weeks of double-blind, double-dummy, placebo-controlled treatment. End points included change from baseline in patient UI symptoms, incontinence-specific quality of life, and safety.

TD-OXY and tolterodine significantly reduced the number of daily incontinence episodes, increased voided volume (Table 1), and significantly improved quality of life (Incontinence Impact

Table 1
Incontinence episodes per day, daily micturition frequency, and average void volume at baseline, end point, and change from baseline among patients taking transdermal oxybutynin, oral extended-release tolterodine, or placebo

Efficacy end points	Transdermal oxybutynin (3.9 mg/d)	Tolterodine (4 mg/d)	Placebo
Incontinence episodes (number/d)[a]			
Baseline	4	4	4
End point	1	1	2
Change	−3	−3	−2
P versus placebo	0.0137	0.0011	—
P versus active comparison	0.5878		
Micturition frequency (number/d)[a]			
Baseline	12	12	12
End point	10	10	10
Change	−2	−2	−1
P versus placebo	0.1010	0.0025	—
P versus active comparison	0.2761		
Average void volume (mL)[a]			
Baseline	160	150	171
End point	188	193	165
Change	24	29	6.5
P versus placebo	0.0023	0.0006	—
P versus active comparison	0.7690		

[a] Median values.

Data from Dmochowski RR, Sand PK, Zinner NR, et al. Comparative efficacy and safety of transdermal oxybutynin and oral tolterodine versus placebo in previously treated patients with urge and mixed urinary incontinence Urology 2003;168:580–6.

Questionnaire total score, $P < 0.05$; Urinary Distress Inventory—Irritative Symptoms subscale, $P < 0.05$) compared with placebo. Pairwise efficacy comparisons between active treatments demonstrated no significant differences ($P > 0.05$). The most common adverse reaction in the OXY group was application-site pruritus (14% versus 4.3% placebo), accompanied by a relatively lower incidence of dry mouth compared with tolterodine (4.1% versus 7.3%, respectively, versus 1.7% for placebo; $P < 0.05$). These data show that TD-OXY produces a level of effectiveness comparable to the most commonly prescribed oral medication for OAB, with a lower incidence of dry mouth.

Safety and tolerability

The most common adverse events for TD-OXY were localized application-site pruritus and erythema. A low incidence of systemic anticholinergic side effects, comparable to that of placebo, was noted in all studies (Table 2). Notably, the incidence of dry mouth was lower than that reported in literature for oral formulations of OXY and was similar to the incidence observed with placebo [8]. The incidence of diarrhea and constipation was not significantly different from placebo.

Local application-site reactions

Local application-site reactions with TD-OXY are generally transient and involve self-limiting, mild-to-moderate pruritus and erythema. Most patients experience no or mild-to-moderate application-site reactions. Of the latter, very few reactions are severe, which require discontinuation. Pruritis appears to be a more troublesome symptom than erythema.

Although no trials have been conducted to compare incidence of application reactions, local tolerability reactions to TD-OXY are generally similar to those of other types of transdermal matrix products [19,20]. Studies of hormone replacement matrix and fentanyl reservoir transdermal systems have revealed higher application-site reaction rates (41%–53%) [21,22].

Because proper use of the product can reduce the chance of developing an application-site reaction, patients should be instructed to apply the system to dry, intact skin on the abdomen, hip, or buttock. A new application site should be selected with each new system to avoid reapplication at the

Table 2
Emergence of adverse events

Adverse event	Transdermal oxybutynin (3.9 mg/d) (n = 125) (%)	Placebo adverse event (n = 132) (%)
Abnormal vision	0	1.5
Constipation	0.8	3.0
Diarrhea	3.2	2.3
Dry mouth	9.6	8.3
Application-site pruritus	16.8	6.1
Application-site erythema	5.6	2.3

Data from Dmochowski RR, Davila GW, Zinner NR, et al. Efficacy and safety of transdermal oxybutynin in patients with urge and mixed urinary incontinence. J Urol 2002;168:580–6.

same site within any 7-day period. Mild erythema may be seen after the patch is removed but generally resolves within a few hours.

Skin tolerability

Topical reactions are a common concern among patients. In a study focusing on skin reactivity, skin tolerability at application sites was evaluated every 3 weeks during the double-blind period and then at 2, 4, and 12 weeks during the open-label period, independent of reported adverse events [23]. Skin tolerability was assessed by visual inspection of the most recently used application site and rated according to a 4-point scale (absent to severe erythema). On study completion, patients completed questionnaires concerning their perception of treatment benefit and their willingness to continue transdermal treatment. Results showed that 86% of patients reported no or mild erythema. The number of days to erythema onset ranged from 29 to 39 days in the double-blind period and from 89 to 133 days during the open-label period. In addition, in most cases, erythema was reversible and minimally perceptible after 24 hours. During the double-blind period, 6.4% of patients withdrew from the trial, whereas 3.4% withdrew during the open-label period because of adverse skin reactions. Pruritis at the application site may occur and be bothersome in up to 16% of patients (Fig. 4); however, rarely is it significant enough to warrant discontinuation of therapy. The discontinuation rate did not correlate with an increase in severity of application-site reactions. Of those who completed the double-blind period, 94% of patients continued to the open-label period. Overall, 66% indicated a preference for transdermal delivery compared with oral or other treatment options. Most skin reactions are temporary, resolving within days of patch removal. If

necessary, skin moisturizers or topical steroid ointments may be used.

A voluntary patient satisfaction questionnaire was completed in which study participants were asked to comment on their experiences with transdermal therapy during the double-blind phase of the study compared with previous oral therapy. The results showed that 67% of patients were satisfied with the appearance of the transdermal system (eg, transparency, discretion) and did not find it bothersome. Sixty-eight percent described the system as easy to apply. Seventy-eight percent of patients found that remembering to reapply the transdermal system was the same or easier than remembering to take a pill each day. Of those patients who completed the questionnaire and who experienced application site itching, most (72%) reported that these symptoms disappeared within a week.

Continuation of treatment

Treatment continuation rates have been high in TD-OXY clinical trials. The initial phase III trial involved a 12-week TD-OXY evaluation, with a 12-week open-label period and an optional 28-week safety extension period [24]. Of the original 520 patients, 86% completed the double-blind period, 92% of eligible patients continued into the open-label period, and 87% of those completed the open-label period [25]. The second phase III trial had similar findings, with 89.9% completing the double-blind phase and 79% enrolling in and 89% completing the open-label period.

The Multicenter Assessment of Transdermal Therapy in Overactive Bladder with Oxybutynin study is a 6-month, open-label, randomized, multicenter, prospective trial in a community-based population. This study is under way to assess safety, health-related quality of life, and other patient-reported outcomes in a large

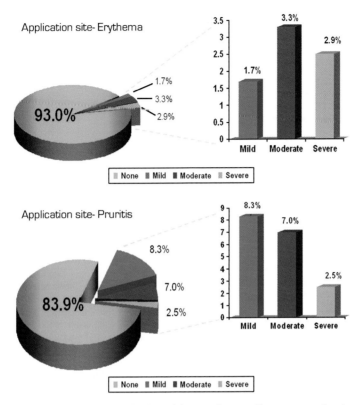

Fig. 4. (*A*) Skin erythema and (*B*) pruritis occur in a small percentage of patients.

number of patients treated with TD-OXY. Study entry data are already being reported and providing useful information regarding the current demographics of the populations of those suffering from OAB [26].

Summary

At a dose of 3.9 mg/d, TD-OXY administered in a twice-weekly regimen is an effective, safe, and well-tolerated treatment for patients who have symptoms of OAB. Efficacy has been demonstrated to be comparable to common treatment regimens: immediate-release OXY in the phase II study, extended-release OXY in the pharmacokinetic study, and tolterodine in the phase III study. OXY plasma levels were stable and correlated with significant median reductions in the number of incontinence episodes and urinary frequency, along with an increase in voided volume, thus providing supporting evidence regarding the efficacy of the transdermal system. Most important, TD-OXY was associated with a low incidence of anticholinergic adverse events, particularly dry mouth, at a rate comparable to placebo. Because the high incidence of such side effects often causes patients to discontinue oral anticholinergics, the data are encouraging. Local application-site reactions were generally mild, involving pruritus and erythema.

The development of a transdermal delivery system for OXY represents a significant improvement in the administration of a drug with a long clinical track record and a high degree of acceptance in the treatment of OAB. Because of its well-recognized anticholinergic side effect profile, the efficacy of oral OXY has been limited in most patients. The alteration in OXY metabolism following transdermal delivery is demonstrated to result in a potentially beneficial alteration in the drug's side effect profile.

The pharmacokinetic data regarding TD-OXY further emphasize the role of the parent compound in achieving a beneficial response regarding OAB symptoms and the role of its metabolites in the development of effect-negating side effects. This clinical observation may prove important in the development of future therapies for the treatment of OAB.

Patch size determines OXY dosage delivered. As such, a dosage requirement of greater than

3.9 mg/d would require a larger patch or multiple patches, possibly increasing the rate of skin reactivity or making this treatment modality financially unsuitable. OXY lends itself to individualization in dosage on a chronic basis and for specific short-term usage. Because transdermal matrix dosing is dependent on patch surface area, many patients have increased their dosage by applying an extra patch or a portion of one [27,28]. The increased circulating OXY level can be expected to improve response rates based on the previous phase II trial data. Other means of increasing circulating OXY include taking an oral dosage. This strategy has been used by taking half or one entire immediate-release tablet immediately before an activity during which OAB symptoms would be particularly undesirable, such as airplane travel or going to a concert or an opera. Rarely has extended-release dosing been used for this purpose.

The use of an effective patch delivery system is well accepted by obstetricians/gynecologists and primary care physicians who are accustomed to other transdermal drug delivery applications. Urologists, on the other hand, are not as familiar with the use of matrix-type patches for drug delivery. Urologists should familiarize themselves with this novel delivery system and become aware of its potential benefits in terms of compliance with therapy due to ease of administration and reduced side effect profile.

Certain subgroups of patients will likely benefit to a greater degree from this drug delivery system. These patients include the elderly and those residing in nursing homes, those who have a neurogenic bladder, and those who have a difficult time taking oral medications. No studies have yet been performed in children, and more studies are required in an adult male population. Future studies will be required to evaluate the use of TD-OXY in these subgroups.

References

[1] Levin RM, Wein AJ. Direct measurement of the anticholinergic activity of a series of pharmacological compounds on the canine and rabbit urinary bladder. J Urol 1982;128:396–8.

[2] Kachur JF, Peterson JS, Carter JP, et al. R and S enantiomers of oxybutynin: pharmacological effects in guinea pig bladder and intestine. J Pharmacol Exp Ther 1988;247:867–72.

[3] Batra S, Biorklund A, Hedlund H, et al. Identification and characterization of muscarinic cholinergic receptors in the human urinary bladder and parotid gland. J Auton Nerv Syst 1987;20:129–35.

[4] Nilvebrant L, Andersson KE, Gillberg PG, et al. Tolterodine: a new bladder-selective antimuscarinic agent. Eur J Pharmacol 1997;327:195–207.

[5] Wang P, Luthin GR, Ruggieri MR. Muscarinic acetylcholine receptor subtypes mediating urinary bladder contractility and coupling to GTP binding proteins. J Pharmacol Exp Ther 1995;273: 959–66.

[6] Nagy F, Hamvas A, Frang D. Idiopathic bladder hyperactivity treated with Ditropan (oxybutynin chloride). Int Urol Nephrol 1990;22:519–24.

[7] Nilvebrant L, Sparf B. Different affinities of some anticholinergic drugs between the parotid gland and ileum. Scand J Gastroenterol 1982;72(Suppl): 69–77.

[8] Anderson RU, Mobley D, Blank B, et al. Once daily controlled versus immediate release oxybutynin chloride for urge urinary incontinence: OROS Oxybutynin Study Group. J Urol 1999;161: 1809–12.

[9] Davila GW, Daugherty CA, Sanders SW. A short-term, multicenter, randomized double-blind dose titration study of the efficacy and anticholinergic side effects of transdermal compared to immediate release oral oxybutynin treatment of patients with urge urinary incontinence. J Urol 2001;166:140–5.

[10] Ranade VV. Drug delivery systems 6. Transdermal drug delivery. J Clin Pharmacol 1991;31:401–18.

[11] Zobrist RH, Schmid B, Feick A, et al. Pharmacokinetics of the R- and S-enantiomers of oxybutynin and N-desethyloxybutynin following oral and transdermal administration of the racemate in healthy volunteers. Pharm Res 2001;18:1029–34.

[12] Verma RK, Garg S. Current status of drug delivery technologies and future directions. Pharm Tech Online 2001;25:1–14.

[13] Bowen AJ, John VA, Ramirez ME, et al. Bioavailability of oestradiol from the Alora™ (0.1 mg/day) oestradiol matrix transdermal delivery system compared with Estraderm™ (0.1 mg/day). J Obstet Gynecol 1998;18:575–80.

[14] Oxytrol package insert. Corona (CA): Watson Pharma, Inc.; 2003.

[15] Zobrist RH, Quan D, Thomas HM, et al. Pharmacokinetics and metabolism of transdermal oxybutynin: in vitro and in vivo performance of a novel delivery system. Pharm Res 2003;20:103–9.

[16] Appell RA, Chancellor M, Zobrist RH, et al. Pharmacokinetics, metabolism, and saliva output during transdermal and extended-release oral oxybutynin administration in healthy subjects. Mayo Clin Proc 2003;78:696–702.

[17] Dmochowski RR, Davila GW, Zinner NR, et al. Efficacy and safety of transdermal oxybutynin in patients with urge and mixed urinary incontinence. J Urol 2002;168(2):580–6.

[18] Dmochowski RR, Sand PK, Zinner NR, et al. Comparative efficacy and safety of transdermal oxybutynin and oral tolterodine versus placebo in previously treated patients with urge and mixed urinary incontinence. Urology 2003;62(2):237–42.

[19] Notelovitz M, Cassel D, Hille D, et al. Efficacy of continuous sequential transdermal estradiol and norethindrone acetate in relieving vasomotor symptoms associated with menopause. Am J Obstet Gynecol 2000;182:7–12.

[20] Weiss SR, Ellman Hdolker M. A randomized controlled trial of four doses of transdermal estradiol for preventing postmenopausal bone loss: Transdermal Estradiol Investigator Group. Obstet Gynecol 1999;94:330–6.

[21] Lopes P, Rozenberg S, Graaf J, et al. Aerodiol versus the transdermal route: perspectives for patient preference. Maturitas 2001;38(Suppl 1):S31–9.

[22] Allan L, Hays H, Jensen NH, et al. Randomised crossover trial of transdermal fentanyl and sustained release oral morphine for treating chronic non-cancer pain. BMJ 2001;322:1154–8.

[23] Newman D.K. Patient perceptions of new therapeutic options for the control of overactive bladder [abstract]. Presented at The Society of Urologic Nurses and Associates. San Antonio, Texas, 2003.

[24] Dmochowski RR, Davila GW, Sanders SW. Transdermal oxybutynin and controlled-release oral tolterodine in patients with positive treatment effect to anticholinergic therapy for overactive bladder [abstract]. Neurourol Urodyn 2002;21:380.

[25] Data on file. Corona (CA): Watson Pharma, Inc.; 2003.

[26] Sand PK, Dmochowski RR, Goldberg RP, et al. Does overactive bladder impact interest in sexual activity: Baseline results from the Matrix study. Int Urogynecol J 2005;16(Suppl 2):S122.

[27] Zinner NR, Davila G, Anderson RP. Dose modulation using oxybutynin transdermal system for overactive bladder in older adults. J Am Geriatr Soc 2004;52(S1):S76–7.

[28] Ruscin JM, Staskin DR, Sand PK, et al. Dose modulation of oxybutynin transdermal system for overactive bladder. Consultant Pharm 2004;19(10):938.

ELSEVIER
SAUNDERS

Urol Clin N Am 33 (2006) 465–473

UROLOGIC
CLINICS
of North America

Trospium Chloride: Distinct Among Other Anticholinergic Agents Available for the Treatment of Overactive Bladder

David R. Staskin, MD

Department of Urology, New York Presbyterian Hospital, Weill-Cornell Medical College,
525 East 68th Street-F9 West, New York, NY 10021, USA

Trospium chloride is an antimuscarinic agent indicated for the treatment of overactive bladder (OAB) with symptoms of urge urinary incontinence, urgency, and urinary frequency. It has been available in Europe for over 20 years and has recently been licensed for use in the United States.

Trospium has three pharmacologic properties that are distinct from other antimuscarinic agents: (1) it is a positively charged quaternary ammonium compound (Fig. 1); (2) it is not metabolized by the cytochrome P-450 (CYP450) system in the liver [1]; and (3) 60% of the absorbed trospium is excreted as the pharmacologically active unchanged parent compound in the urine [2]. Other currently available compounds are tertiary amines metabolized by the CYP450 system and excreted unchanged or as active metabolites in small quantities.

Clinical studies

The availability of trospium for over 2 decades in Europe has resulted in a wealth of efficacy and safety data, derived from over 20 clinical trials and postsurveillance marketing studies involving over 10,000 patients [3]. These data indicate that trospium provides effective relief for the troublesome symptoms of OAB and that safety is not limited by significant side effects such as dry mouth or central nervous system (CNS) adverse events.

More recently, two phase III clinical trials of trospium have been performed in the United States [4,5]. The results of these studies are of particular interest because unlike the European studies, to be eligible for inclusion, patients were not required to have urodynamically confirmed detrusor instability. Instead, inclusion criteria were based on the presence of symptoms of OAB: urinary urgency, voiding frequency, and urge incontinence. The role for urodynamic assessment in the diagnosis of OAB is controversial because urodynamically detectable detrusor overactivity may not be present in up to 25% of patients who have OAB symptoms, and patients who have the condition appear to respond equally well to antimuscarinic therapy regardless of whether their symptoms are urodynamically verified [6]. In 2002, the International Continence Society (ICS) redefined OAB based on symptoms (specifically, urgency) rather than on urodynamic parameters [7]. Because the two United States studies most closely represent the updated definition of OAB, the results from these studies form the body of this review.

Treatment with trospium chloride provides significant improvements in frequency, volume voided, and urge incontinence episodes

The United States studies were 12-week, multicenter, placebo-controlled trials involving 1157 patients that aimed to determine the effects of trospium given as 20-mg tablets versus placebo twice daily [4,5]. To qualify for participation in the studies, patients had to meet the following inclusion criteria: urge or mixed incontinence (with a predominance of urge), at least seven urge incontinence episodes per week, and a minimum voiding frequency of 70 voids per week. Patients

E-mail address: das2021@med.cornell.edu

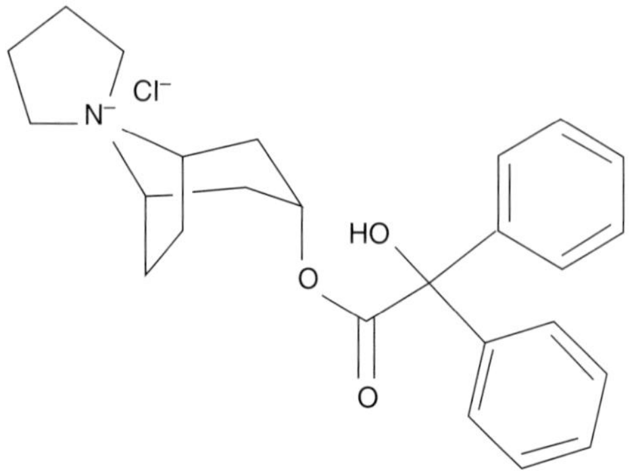

Fig. 1. Quaternary amine structure of trospium chloride.

who had incontinence that was predominantly stress, insensate, or overflow in nature were excluded, as were those who had neurogenic disorders. After 12 weeks of treatment with trospium, significant improvements were observed compared with placebo in all of the key parameters commonly used to asses the efficacy of OAB medications: urinary frequency, urge incontinence episodes, and urinary void volume (Table 1).

Patients' perceptions of urgency are significantly improved following treatment with trospium chloride

A key measure included in both of the United States trials was the validated Indevus Urgency Severity Scale (IUSS), a 4-point validated scale

rating patients' perceptions of urgency severity at each void [8]. Urgency, as defined by the ICS, is the keystone symptom of OAB and has a significant negative effect on patients' health-related quality of life [9]. It should be noted that the IUSS scale uses "urge to void" as opposed to "desire to void," unlike the strict ICS definition [9]. Indeed, urgency is often the symptom that prompts patients to seek help, yet in many studies evaluating OAB therapies, measures of treatment success have been limited to changes in parameters such as frequency of urgency episodes rather than the severity of urgency episodes. In both studies, trospium significantly decreased the average urgency severity at each void (Fig. 2). The reduction in IUSS score was significant in both studies after only 1 week of treatment with trospium compared with placebo. It was concluded that patients receiving trospium moved from having a moderate degree of urgency with each toilet void toward experiencing milder sensations of urgency during the treatment period.

Improvements provided by trospium chloride are clinically meaningful as measured by the Overactive Bladder Symptom Composite Score

There are additional factors that may influence the sensation of urgency that patients feel at each void. Many patients will void when the opportunity arises—for example, when

Table 1

Mean change from baseline to end of treatment[a] for urinary frequency, urge incontinence episodes, and void volume in two United States Phase III studies

	Study 1 [4]			Study 2 [5]		
Efficacy end point	Placebo (n = 256)	Trospium (n = 253)	P	Placebo (n = 325)	Trospium (n = 323)	P
Urinary frequency/24 h[b,c]						
Baseline	12.9	12.7		13.2	12.9	
Change from baseline	−1.29	−2.37	≤0.0001	−1.76	−2.67	<0.0001
Urge incontinence episodes/24 h[b,d]						
Baseline	4.3	3.9		2.86	2.86	
Change from baseline	−44.2	−59.0	≤0.0001	−1.29	−1.86	<0.0001
Urinary void volume/toilet void/24 h (mL)						
Baseline	156.6	155.1		154.6	154.8	
Change from baseline	7.7	32.1	≤0.0001	9.44	35.59	<0.0001

[a] End of treatment was week 1 or last observation carried forward.

[b] Denotes coprimary endpoint for Study 1.

[c] Denotes primary end point for study 2.

[d] Difference assessed by rank analysis of variance; all others assessed by analysis of variance.

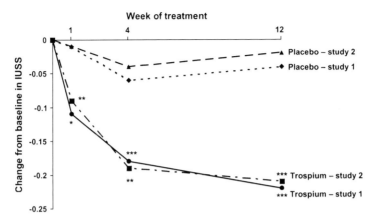

Fig. 2. Mean change from baseline in the IUSS score by visit in two United States placebo-controlled studies. (*Data from* Zinner N, Gittelman M, Harris R, et al. Trospium chloride improves overactive bladder symptoms: a multicenter phase III trial. J Urol 2004;171:2311–5; and Rudy D, Cline K, Harris R, et al. Multicenter phase III trial studying trospium chloride in patients with overactive bladder. Urology 2006;67(2):275–80.)

passing a toilet—rather than when they have the urge to do so. This practice may decrease the average urgency severity per toilet void but may increase the frequency of toilet voids per day. To understand fully the clinical importance of the reduction in urgency, data from the United States trials were pooled and a combined suite of OAB symptoms was examined [10]. The OAB Symptom Composite Score (OAB-SCS) comprises common patient-reported diary data including 24-hour voiding frequency, urgency severity associated with each toilet void, and the frequency of each urge urinary incontinence episode. An important feature of the OAB-SCS is that it does not count all voids equally. Instead, the OAB-SCS assigns a single quantifiable value to the overall number and severity of OAB

symptoms, taking into account the association between voiding frequency and urgency severity, and accounts for incontinence episodes whether or not the patient completely voids the bladder and is unable to reach a toilet [10].

Analysis of data from the two pooled United States studies revealed a significant reduction in the OAB-SCS for trospium compared with placebo at each time point recorded (Fig. 3) [10]. These reductions reflect an improvement based on the three primary symptoms of OAB and the associations between these symptoms.

Stratification of the results according to baseline OAB-SCS, which can be approximately equated to patients having mild, moderate, or severe OAB symptoms, indicated that improvements of a similar magnitude were observed

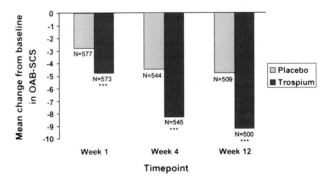

Fig. 3. Mean change from baseline in OAB-SCS in the intent to treat population (observed cases data). (*From* Zinner N, Harnett M, Sabounjian L, et al. The Overactive Bladder–Symptom Composite Score: a composite symptom score of toilet voids, urgency severity and urge urinary incontinence in patients with overactive bladder. J Urol 2005;173:1641; with permission from the American Urological Association.)

irrespective of the baseline severity of the disease (Fig. 4) [10]. After 12 weeks of treatment, the mean change from baseline in the trospium and placebo groups, respectively, was 5 and 1 OAB-SCS points in patients who had mild OAB, 10 and 5 in patients who had moderate OAB, and 13 and 9 in patients who had severe OAB. The design of the OAB-SCS allows any change in the score to be directly translated into a number of combinations of voids of varying severity or incontinence episodes. This design permits clinically relevant interpretations of decreases in the OAB-SCS to be derived. For example, from baseline to week 12, the difference between trospium-treated patients and those receiving placebo was 5 OAB-SCS points. This average change can be viewed as clinically equivalent to, for example, (1) an average group daily decrease of more than three moderate urgency toilet voids; (2) an average group daily decrease of two severe urgency toilet voids; or (3) an average group daily decrease of two urge urinary incontinence episodes [10].

Overall, the results indicate that treatment with trospium provides clinically meaningful improvements in OAB symptoms. The analyses were, however, performed after the clinical trials were completed, and further verification of the OAB-SCS in a future trial of trospium would be beneficial.

Treatment with trospium chloride separates from placebo by day 3

Data from the two United States studies have been further analyzed to examine the onset of action of trospium in terms of reducing the symptoms of OAB within the first week of treatment [11,12]. Treatment with trospium was associated with a significant reduction in daily void frequency and urge urinary incontinence episodes compared with placebo within the first 7 days of treatment. For the reduction in daily void frequency, separation from placebo was seen as early as day 3 of treatment in one study [11] and from day 5 onward in the other study [12]. Rudy and coworkers [12] also reported a significant reduction in the severity of urgency symptoms ($P = 0.015$ versus placebo) from day 3 onward [12]. A further subanalysis of these data in female patients who had OAB also confirmed a significant reduction in daily void frequency ($P = 0.0063$), urge incontinence episodes ($P < 0.0001$), and urgency severity ($P < 0.0001$) after 1 week of treatment among patients treated with trospium compared with those who received placebo [13].

Symptomatic improvements following treatment with trospium chloride are paralleled by improvements in patient-perceived quality-of-life measures

In the Zinner and colleagues' [4] study, quality of life and symptom annoyance were measured using the Incontinence Impact Questionnaire (IIQ), which has subscales that measure the impact of OAB on travel, physical activity, social relationships, and emotional health. After 12 weeks, total IIQ scores had significantly improved for all women treated with trospium compared with placebo ($P \leq 0.05$). Trospium had a significant effect

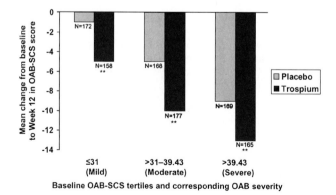

Fig. 4. Mean change from baseline in OAB-SCS at week 12 by baseline tertile groupings in the intent to treat population (observed cases data). (*From* Zinner N, Harnett M, Sabounjian L, et al. The Overactive Bladder–Symptom Composite Score: a composite symptom score of toilet voids, urgency severity and urge urinary incontinence in patients with overactive bladder. J Urol 2005;173:1641; with permission from the American Urological Association.)

on the IIQ subscales of emotional health, social relationships, and travel, and improvements were seen in specific items such as sleep, feelings of anxiety, feelings of frustration and embarrassment, the way patients dressed, fear of odor, and travel to unfamiliar places. In men, the IIQ did not show significant improvement, but because the IIQ scale was not validated in men, it may have been an inappropriate measure to have used [4].

Trospium chloride is well tolerated, with discontinuation rates similar to placebo

Tolerability is an important concern for patients taking anticholinergic medication. The unpleasant side effects of dry mouth and constipation often limit the usefulness of these agents. Patients may take less than optimal doses in an attempt to reduce the incidence or severity of the side effects, and some patients may stop taking the medication altogether.

In the two United States studies, the treatment discontinuation rates due to adverse events ranged from 7.6% to 8.8% and were similar to the discontinuation rates observed with placebo (4.9% to 5.7%) [4,5]. In all of the placebo-controlled trials combined, the incidence of serious adverse events was 2.9% with trospium (20-mg twice daily) and 1.5% with placebo. Of these events, 0.2% and 0.3% were judged to be at least possibly related to treatment with trospium and placebo, respectively. Treatment with trospium was associated with a higher incidence of dry mouth (20.1% versus 5.8%) and constipation (9.6% versus 4.6%) than placebo in these two studies [14]. Dry mouth led to discontinuation in only 1.9% of patients treated with trospium.

CNS adverse events associated with trospium were not seen or were seen only at low rates and were comparable to placebo: blurred vision (0.0% with trospium versus 0.8% with placebo), daytime somnolence (0.3% with trospium versus 0.2% with placebo), dizziness (1.5% with trospium versus 1.0% with placebo), and anxiety (0.2% with trospium versus 0.0% with placebo) [14].

Although the incidence of CNS adverse events is dependent on the individual patient, a number of studies have shown that CNS adverse events with trospium therapy do not differ from those with placebo. Staskin and Harnett [15] specifically investigated the effects of trospium on CNS adverse events and on daytime sleepiness using the Stanford Sleepiness Scale. In this placebo-controlled study, the incidence of spontaneous CNS adverse events among patients receiving trospium was low and similar to the placebo group (5.8% versus 5.2%, respectively), and there were no clinically relevant changes in the Stanford Sleepiness Scale for patients taking trospium. Diefenbach and colleagues [16] examined the effects of trospium, oxybutynin, and tolterodine on sleep and cognitive skills in healthy volunteers. After treatment with trospium, rapid eye movement (REM) sleep latency and duration were comparable with placebo. This result was in contrast to the effects observed with oxybutynin and tolterodine, both of which resulted in a significant reduction in REM sleep of approximately 15% and a slightly (but not significantly) greater REM latency compared with placebo. None of the anticholinergic agents tested had any effect on cognitive and subjective sleep variables.

Pharmacology

The quaternary amine trospium chloride theoretically should not cross the blood-brain barrier

The distribution of anticholinergic agents—in particular, their ability to penetrate the CNS—is a key consideration in their safety. Transfer of anticholinergic agents into the CNS is known to cause serious anticholinergic side effects such as changes in memory, disruption of sleep, hallucinations, confusion, and delirium.

As a quaternary amine, trospium has low lipophilicity and is charged at neutral pH. These factors limit passive transfer of this compound across lipid membranes including those of the blood-brain barrier [1]. Although there have been no studies directly measuring trospium levels in cerebrospinal fluid in humans, studies in rats indicate that passage across the blood-brain barrier is very low [1]. Indirect data supporting a lack of CNS penetration in humans are available from experimental studies, clinical studies, postmarketing surveillance data, and physician experience [14–18]. For example, the CNS effects of three antimuscarinic agents (oxybutynin, tolterodine, and trospium) were examined in a study of healthy adult men. Following administration of the recommended daily doses, it was found that oxybutynin caused significant quantitative-topographic electroencephalograph power reductions in four frequency bands, whereas trospium and tolterodine did not [18]. The clinical significance of these results is unclear; however, the findings provide an indication of the ability of different agents to enter the CNS.

The relative ranking of available antimuscarinic agents for the treatment of OAB for lipophilicity and potential ease in crossing the blood-brain barrier is predicted to be highest for darifenacin compared with oxybutynin/solifenacin, lower for tolterodine, and lowest for trospium [19,20]. This may affect their relative safety, particularly with respect to CNS anticholinergic adverse effects.

The low lipophilicity of trospium also limits transfer of this compound across the lipid membranes of the gastrointestinal tract [2]. Following oral administration of trospium to healthy volunteers, less than 10% of the dose is absorbed by the gastrointestinal tract, with peak plasma levels of trospium reached at 4 to 5 hours after administration of a 20-mg immediate-release preparation [2]. The low absorption of trospium contributes to a low bioavailability (9.6% for trospium [20 mg] compared with 15% for darifenacin [7.5 mg] and >90% for solifenacin [10 mg]) [2,21,22], but because it is possible to increase the absorbed amount of trospium by increasing the dose and because the unabsorbed compound does not result in adverse events, bioavailability per se may not be the most appropriate means by which to compare agents.

No clinically relevant cytochrome P-450–mediated drug–drug interactions are anticipated with trospium chloride

When evaluating the metabolism of a compound, it is imperative to consider the site of its metabolism, the metabolic pathway used, and whether any active metabolites are produced because these factors may influence the incidence of adverse events and the potential for adverse drug–drug interactions. This potential is especially relevant in the elderly, who are prone to polypharmacy [23,24]. Trospium is metabolized by way of a hepatic esterase, and most of the absorbed fraction of trospium is excreted unchanged in the urine. A small fraction appears as the spiroalcohol, a metabolite formed by ester hydrolysis [2]. An important consequence of this metabolic process is that trospium is not a substrate or an inhibitor of the hepatic CYP450 enzyme system. Metabolic studies of trospium incubated with isolated human hepatic microsomes showed minimal CYP450 metabolism and no inhibitory effects on CYP3A4, CYP2D6, CYP1A2, CYP2E1, CYP2C19, CYP2C9, and CYP2A6 isoenzymes at clinical dose levels (inhibitory concentration of 50% >1 μmol) [1]. Based on these in vitro data, no clinically relevant drug–drug

interactions related to the metabolism of trospium are expected [2].

As tertiary amines, all of the other antimuscarinic agents available for the treatment of OAB are metabolized by way of the CYP450 enzymes of the liver, and consideration should therefore be given to the possibility of interactions between these agents and other drugs metabolized by way of the same hepatic CYP450 pathways.

Metabolism independent of the CYP450 system also means that the bioavailability of trospium is less affected by the genetic differences in metabolism that are present in the general population. Up to 10% of the Caucasian population are devoid of the CYP2D6 metabolic pathway, resulting in increased exposure to agents that are metabolized in this way. The bioavailability of tolterodine, which is metabolized by CYP2D6, ranges from 91% in poor metabolizers to 26% among extensive metabolizers [25]. Because trospium is not metabolized by way of this pathway, exposure is not altered in poor metabolizers.

Excretion of active trospium chloride by way of the kidneys may provide additional benefits by way of afferent pathways

For compounds that are extensively metabolized and then excreted in an inactive form, the pathway by which they are eliminated may be of little interest. For trospium, however, the excretory pathway is of particular interest because it may underlie some of the efficacy (particularly in terms of rapid onset of action and effect on urgency) that is observed with this compound.

After it is absorbed, trospium is predominantly excreted through the kidneys, [1,26] with 60%–80% of the absorbed dose excreted as unchanged compound [2]. The high percentage of activity of trospium in urine contrasts that of other anticholinergic agents, whose activity in urine ranges from 0.1% to 11% of absorbed compound (Table 2).

Excretion of trospium in the active form may provide additional and prolonged efficacy because the active molecules could bathe the mucosal muscarinic receptors of the bladder urothelium during the bladder urine storage phase. The clinical validity for a local "topical" rather than systemic effect of antimuscarinic agents has recently been demonstrated using intravesical instillation of human urine, collected following oral ingestion of trospium, tolterodine, or oxybutynin, into the bladders of rats. As predicted by measurable activity in human urine, trospium had

Table 2
Active drug, active metabolite, or both excreted in urine[a]

	Trospium (%)	Oxybutynin (%)	Tolterodine (%)	Darifenacin (%)	Solifenacin (%)
Unchanged compound	60–80	<0.1	<1	1.8	<10.3
Active metabolite	0	0	3.9–10.8	0	0

[a] Values are the percentage of the absorbed dose excreted in the urine as calculated from product prescribing information.

Data from Refs. [14,22,34–36].

a significant effect on carbachol-induced bladder overactivity in the rat bladder [27]. The same effect was not seen for oxybutynin or tolterodine, which may reflect their extensive hepatic metabolism and thus lower activity in urine.

The mean renal clearance for trospium is fourfold higher than the average glomerular filtration rate, suggesting that tubular secretion is an additional route of elimination. Because tubular secretion is an active process, there have been theoretic concerns that there may be pharmacokinetic interactions with other drugs eliminated by active tubular secretion (eg, digoxin, procainamide, vancomycin, and metformin). A recent study designed specifically to evaluate the potential interaction between trospium and digoxin found that neither drug influenced the pharmacologic profile of the other, suggesting that competitive inhibition with other agents excreted by active tubular secretion may not be a concern with trospium [28].

Preclinical pharmacology

Muscarinic receptor inhibition

The question as to which muscarinic subtypes are involved in mediating contraction of the lower urinary tract has received significant attention in recent years because of the potential for using selective muscarinic antagonists in the treatment of OAB. Receptor immunoprecipitation studies have identified the presence of the M_2 and the M_3 receptor subtypes in detrusor smooth muscle; however, the M_2 receptor subtypes outnumber the M_3 receptors by a ratio of approximately 3:1 [29]. Despite the predominance of the M_2 receptors, evidence suggests that the M_3 receptors are most important for direct activation of detrusor smooth muscle contraction, whereas M_2 receptors appear to block β-adrenergic receptor–mediated detrusor smooth muscle relaxation, thereby facilitating cholinergic contraction [29,30].

Receptor-binding studies have shown that trospium is a broad-spectrum antimuscarinic agent with similar high affinity for the M_1, M_2, M_3, M_4, and M_5 subtypes of muscarinic receptors [31] and that the agent has negligible affinity for nicotinic receptors compared with muscarinic receptors at concentrations similar to those found at therapeutic doses [14].

Selectivity for the M_3 muscarinic receptor has been proposed as a mechanism by which antimuscarinic agents provide clinical efficacy for the treatment of OAB while minimizing the incidence of adverse effects and safety issues related to blockade of other muscarinic receptor subtypes [32]. It is suggested that sparing the M_1 and M_2 receptors would limit the incidence of cognitive and cardiac adverse effects, respectively. It is unfortunate, however, that M_3 receptors are found in the gut and salivary glands in addition to the bladder, and thus the incidence of dry mouth and constipation would not be reduced by M_3 selectivity. In addition, the M_2 muscarinic receptor takes on an increased role in certain disease states [33], suggesting that in these individuals, pure inhibition of M_3 would not be advisable. The theoretic advantages of M_3 selectivity have yet to be clinically proved [32].

In the case of trospium, the reduced ability to cross the blood-brain barrier (as a consequence of its quaternary amine structure) limits the likelihood of centrally mediated adverse events, irrespective of the muscarinic subtypes present in the CNS.

Summary

Trospium is efficacious in improving the key symptoms of OAB, including reducing daily urge incontinence episodes and daily toilet voids and increasing the volume of urine voided per toilet void. Patients' perceptions of urgency severity at each void are also improved following treatment with trospium, which is an important finding because the experience of urgency has a major effect on patients' health-related quality of life and is often the symptom that initially prompts patients to seek treatment.

As a quaternary amine compound, trospium does not readily cross the blood-brain barrier, a feature that may be especially beneficial among elderly patients who can be susceptible to central anticholinergic effects and who may already be taking other cholinergic drugs, thereby increasing their overall cholinergic load.

Because trospium is not a substrate or an inhibitor of the family of CYP450 isoenzymes or an inhibitor, it is not likely to interfere with other drugs metabolized by those isoenzymes. To date, there have been no known reports of clinically relevant drug interactions with trospium. The absorbed portion of the drug is principally excreted through the kidneys, of which 60% is unchanged, active parent drug. The presence of the active compound in the urine may provide additional and prolonged efficacy because the drug can bathe the muscarinic receptors of the urothelium, providing local effects.

Concerns that trospium might interfere with other drugs that are excreted by way of the same pathway have recently been addressed in a study examining the potential effects of trospium on digoxin transport. In this study, neither drug affected the pharmacokinetic profile of the other, suggesting that concerns regarding competition by way of the renal pathway are unfounded.

These pharmacologic properties underlie the salutary safety and tolerability profile of trospium chloride that has been seen in clinical trials and during postmarketing experience. The lack of CNS adverse events and the ability to coprescribe trospium without concern for interactions with other agents may make trospium the antimuscarinic of choice in certain populations, particularly the elderly.

References

[1] Beckmann-Knopp S, Rietbrock S, Weyhenmeyer R, et al. Inhibitory effects of trospium chloride on cytochrome P450 enzymes in human liver microsomes. Pharmacol Toxicol 1999;85:299–304.

[2] Doroshyenko O, Jetter A, Odenthal KP, et al. Clinical pharmacokinetics of trospium chloride. Clin Pharmacokinet 2005;44:701–20.

[3] Höfner K, Oelke M, Machtens S, et al. Trospium chloride—an effective drug in the treatment of overactive bladder and detrusor hyperreflexia. World J Urol 2001;19:336–43.

[4] Zinner N, Gittelman M, Harris R, et al. Trospium chloride improves overactive bladder symptoms: a multicenter phase III trial. J Urol 2004;171:2311–5.

[5] Rudy D, Cline K, Harris R, et al. Multicenter phase III trial studying trospium chloride in patients with overactive bladder. Urology 2006;67(2):275–80.

[6] Malone-Lee J, Henshaw DJ, Cummings K. Urodynamic verification of an overactive bladder is not a prerequisite for antimuscarinic treatment response. BJU Int 2003;92:415–7.

[7] Abrams P, Cardozo L, Fall M, et al. The standardisation of terminology in lower urinary tract function: report from the standardisation sub-committee of the International Continence Society. Urology 2003; 61:37–49.

[8] Nixon A, Colman S, Sabounjian L, et al. A validated patient reported measure of urinary urgency severity in overactive bladder for use in clinical trials. J Urol 2005;174:604–7.

[9] Coyne KS, Payne C, Bhattacharyya SK, et al. The impact of urinary urgency and frequency on health-related quality of life in overactive bladder: results from a national community survey. Value Health 2004;7:455–63.

[10] Zinner N, Harnett M, Sabounjian L, et al. The Overactive Bladder–Symptom Composite Score: a composite symptom score of toilet voids, urgency severity and urge urinary incontinence in patients with overactive bladder. J Urol 2005;173:1639–43.

[11] Sand P, Dmochowski R. Trospium chloride improves the symptoms of overactive bladder within one week. Presented at the International Continence Society Meeting. Florence, Italy, 2003. Abstract #370.

[12] Rudy D, Cline K, Harris R, et al. Time to onset of improvement in symptoms of overactive bladder using antimuscarinic treatment. BJU Int 2006; 97(3):540–6.

[13] Garely A, for the Trospium Study Group. Trospium chloride demonstrates rapid onset of effect for multiple overactive bladder symptoms in female patients. J Pelvic Med Surg 2005;11(Suppl 1):S41.

[14] Odyssey Pharmaceutical Inc. and Indevus Pharmaceuticals Inc. Sanctura™ prescribing information. July 2004. Available at: www.sanctura.com. Accessed April 1, 2006.

[15] Staskin DR, Harnett MD. Effect of trospium chloride on somnolence and sleepiness in patients with overactive bladder. Curr Sci 2004;5:423–6.

[16] Diefenbach K, Arnold G, Wollny A, et al. Effects on sleep of anticholinergics used for overactive bladder treatment in healthy volunteers aged ≥ 50 years. BJU Int 2005;95:346–9.

[17] Pietzko A, Dimpfel W, Schwantes U, et al. Influences of trospium chloride and oxybutynin on quantitative EEG in healthy volunteers. Eur J Clin Pharmacol 1994;47:337–43.

[18] Todorova A, Vonderheid-Guth B, Dimpfel W. Effects of tolterodine, trospium chloride and oxybutynin on the central nervous system. J Clin Pharmacol 2001;41:636–44.

[19] Pak RW, Petrou SP, Staskin DR. Trospium chloride: a quaternary amine with unique pharmacologic properties. Curr Urol Rep 2003;4:436–40.

[20] Scheife R, Takeda M. Central nervous system safety of anticholinergic drugs for the treatment of overactive bladder in the elderly. Clin Ther 2005;27:144–53.

[21] Kerbusch T, Wahlby U, Milligan PA, et al. Population pharmacokinetic modelling of darifenacin and its hydroxylated metabolite using pooled data, incorporating saturable first-pass metabolism, CYP2D6 genotype and formulation-dependent bioavailability. Br J Clin Pharmacol 2003;56:639–52.

[22] Astellas Pharma US Inc. and GlaxoSmithKline. VES-Icare® prescribing information. November 2004. Available at: www.vesicare.com/assets/vesicare_prescribing_info.pdf. Accessed April 1, 2006.

[23] Kroenke K, Pinholt EM. Reducing polypharmacy in the elderly. A controlled trial of physician feedback. J Am Geriatr Soc 1990;38:31–6.

[24] Brazeau S. Polypharmacy and the elderly. Can J CME 2001;Aug:85–94.

[25] Brynne N, Dalen P, Alvan G, et al. Influence of CYP2D6 polymorphism on the pharmacokinetics and pharmacodynamic of tolterodine. Clin Pharmacol Ther 1998;63:529–39.

[26] Fusgen I, Hauri D. Trospium chloride: an effective option for medical treatment of bladder overactivity. Int J Clin Pharmacol Ther 2000;38:223–34.

[27] Kim Y, Yoshimura N, Masuda H, et al. Intravesical instillation of human urine after oral administration of trospium, tolterodine and oxybutynin in a rat model of detrusor overactivity. BJU Int 2006;97:400–3.

[28] Sandage B, Sabounjian L, Shipley J, et al. Predictive power of an in vitro system to assess drug interactions of an antimuscarinic medication: a comparison of in vitro and in vivo drug-drug interaction studies of trospium chloride with digoxin. J Clin Pharmacol 2006;46(7):776–84.

[29] Wang P, Luthin GR, Ruggieri MR. Muscarinic acetylcholine receptor subtypes mediating urinary bladder contractility and coupling to GTP binding proteins. J Pharmacol Exp Ther 1995;273:959–66.

[30] Hegde SS, Eglen RM. Muscarinic receptor subtypes modulating smooth muscle contractility in the urinary bladder. Life Sci 1999;64:419–28.

[31] Napier C, Gupta P. Darifenacin is selective for the human recombinant M3 receptor subtype. Neurourol Urodyn 2002;21:A445.

[32] Andersson KE. Potential benefits of muscarinic M_3 receptor selectivity. Eur Urol 2002;(Suppl 1): 23–8.

[33] Pontari MA, Braverman AS, Ruggieri MR Sr. The M2 muscarinic receptor mediates in vitro bladder contractions from patients with neurogenic bladder dysfunction. Am J Physiol Regul Integr Comp Physiol 2004;286:R874–80.

[34] Ortho-McNeil Pharmaceutical, Inc. Ditropan XL prescribing information. June 2003. Available at: www.orthomcneil.com/products/pi/pdfs/ditropanxl.pdf. Accessed April 1, 2006.

[35] Pharmacia and Upjohn Company. Detrol® LA prescribing information. April 2004. Available at: www.detrolla.com/files/DetrolLA.pdf. Accessed April 1, 2006.

[36] Novartis Pharmaceuticals Inc. Enablex® prescribing information. December 2004. Available at: http://www.enablex.com/content/prescribing.jsp. Accessed April 1, 2006.

**ELSEVIER
SAUNDERS**

Urol Clin N Am 33 (2006) 475–482

**UROLOGIC
CLINICS
of North America**

Darifenacin: Pharmacology and Clinical Usage

William D. Steers, MD, FACS

*Department of Urology, University of Virginia School of Medicine, University of Virginia Health System,
Box 800422 Hospital Drive, Charlottesville, VA 22908, USA*

Darifenacin is one of several recently approved antimuscarinics for the treatment of overactive bladder and urge urinary incontinence. Darifenacin is manufactured by Novartis, acquired from Pfizer in March 2003. It received Food and Drug Administration approval for the treatment of the overactive bladder (OAB) in December 2004 and was launched in early 2005. Several large prospective, placebo-controlled, randomized clinical trials have demonstrated efficacy for the symptoms of OAB characterized by urgency, usually with frequency and nocturia, with or without urge urinary incontinence [1]. Among the approved muscarinic receptor antagonists, darifenacin has the greatest affinity for the M_3 subtype. This distinguishing pharmacology confers some distinct clinical characteristics for this drug with respect to potential side effects. Whether this confers any advantage in terms of efficacy for OAB relative to other antimuscarinic agents has yet to be demonstrated. This review describes the role of M_3 receptors and covers the mechanism of action, pharmacokinetic properties, clinical efficacy safety and tolerability, drug interactions, and dosing guidelines for darifenacin.

Mechanism of action and role of M_3 muscarinic receptors in micturition

Acetylcholine is the primary neurotransmitter responsible for bladder contraction during normal voiding [2]. Acetylcholine acts at a variety of muscarinic and nicotinic receptors within the bladder and along the neuraxis involved in micturition. There are five muscarinic receptor subtypes, abbreviated M_1, M_2, M_3, M_4, and M_5 [3]. A large

body of evidence indicates that the M_3 receptor expressed by detrusor smooth muscle in the urinary bladder mediates normal contraction during voiding. The human detrusor expresses predominately the M_2 receptor, yet contraction accompanying voiding is probably a result of binding of acetylcholine to the M_3 subtype [4–7]. In a recent study using human detrusor tissue, darifenacin primarily inhibited carbachol (muscarinic agonist)-induced contraction by turning off calcium entry through nifedipine sensitive Ca^{+2} channels and rho kinase rather than through intracellular Ca^{+2} release from intracellular stores [8]. This finding indicates that bladder contraction from activation of the M_3 receptor relies principally on extracellular Ca^{+2}. Human urothelium also contains three times as much mRNA for M_2 as the M_3 receptor [9]. The clinical significance of the M_2 receptor is unclear because transgenic mice with loss of expression of the M_2 receptor void to completion, whereas M_3 knockout mice have large distended bladders [10,11]. Muscarinic receptors also influence bladder tone during filling because acetylcholinesterase inhibitors raise filling pressures, and the nonselective antimuscarinic oxybutynin reduces filling pressures and raises capacity [12].

It is hotly debated what role non-M_3 muscarinic receptors play in normal bladder sensation, filling pressures, and detrusor contractions. Even more unclear is the clinical relevance of M_3 receptor with micturition or incontinence due to aging, denervation, obstruction, inflammation, and other disorders. Whether M_3 blockade is more or less efficacious in subpopulations in a comparator trial has not been examined in sufficient detail to make conclusions. For example, with aging, there is a decline in M_3 but not M_2 receptor mRNA in the human detrusor [9]. In human detrusor tissue

E-mail address: wds6t@virginia.edu

obtained from patients who have neurogenic bladders (spinal cord injury, myelomeningocele), the M_2 receptor mediated bladder contraction [13]. Following hypertrophy of the rat bladder in response to increased outlet resistance, a similar shift from M_3-mediated to M_2-mediated detrusor contraction and a reduction in M_3 receptor density occurs [14]. In streptozotocin-induced diabetic rats, however, an up-regulation of mRNA for M_3 receptor occurs [15]. In a recent animal study, chemical cystitis raised levels of mRNA for the M_5 receptor expressed by urothelium. Furthermore, muscarinic receptors in the central nervous system can influence voiding in animal experiments. Intracerebroventricularly administered darifenacin had no effect on cystometry in the rat, but oxybutynin and tolterodine reduced micturition pressures and raised micturition volumes [16]. Thus, if one believes that the blockade of muscarinic receptors on urothelium (M_2, M_3, M_5), afferents (M_1, M_2, M_3), efferent nerves (M_1, M_2, M_5, N), ganglia, interstitial cells, or both receptors expressed by the detrusor (M_2/M_3) influences symptoms of OAB, then nonselective antimuscarinic drugs should possess greater efficacy. Conversely, if M_3 blockade is crucial for involuntary detrusor contractions and if these contractions are primarily responsible for OAB symptoms, then raising doses of an M_3 selective antagonist should confer the greatest efficacy and the fewest side effects due to actions at muscarinic receptors elsewhere. Effects at sites other than the bladder are also dependent on the pharmacokinetic and biophysical properties of the drug. Using cystometry in rats to gauge relative potencies of antimuscarinics, investigators found that atropine, tolterodine, and oxybutynin reduced carbachol-induced micturition contractions to a greater degree than darifenacin [17]. Although pharmacokinetic and species differences may underlie these findings, they suggest that a higher affinity for M_3 in and of itself does not confer greater potency at reducing voiding contractions.

M_3 receptors are also involved in the contraction of gastrointestinal smooth muscle, the production of saliva, and the control of iris sphincter function. The blurred vision occasionally reported with antimuscarinics is attributed to action on the smooth muscle of the iris. The colon has sixfold more M_2 receptor mRNA than M_3 receptor mRNA [18]. In examining colonic contractions due to the muscarinic agonist carbachol, darifenacin and atropine were equally potent and

exceeded oxybutynin and propantheline [18]. Furthermore, in M_3 knockout mice, no colonic abnormalities have been noted [10].

In the salivary glands, serous cells express M_3 receptors, whereas mucus cells express M_2 and M_3 receptors [19]. Both cell types contribute to dry mouth after darifenacin ingestion. An in vivo study in animals showed darifenacin reduced salivation to a greater extent than agents that were more M_2 selective [20]. Clinically, however, a comparator trial of darifenacin to oxybutynin revealed that the M_3-selective drug had less effect on salivary flow [21]. In other exocrine glands, M_3 and M_2 receptors control secretion.

In the myocardium, only M_2 receptors influence heart rate in response to stimulation of the vagus nerve [22]. Consistent with this latter observation, darifenacin does not prolong the QT/QTc interval or alter heart rate in multiple dosing studies [23]. At very high doses in dogs, darifenacin can shorten the action potential duration, possibly through inhibition of Ca^{+2}, and can reduce the amplitude due to nonselective sodium channel blockade. Of interest, recent data suggest that there may be a functional role for M_3 receptors in the human heart, especially in disease states [24].

Pharmacology of darifenacin

Chemically, darifenacin hydrobromide ($C_{28}H_{30}N_2O_2$·HBR) is (s)-2-{1-[2-(2.3-dihydrobenzofuran-5-yl) ethyl]-3-pyrrolindinyl}-2,2-diphenylacetamide bromide (Fig. 1). It is a white crystalline powder with a molecular weight of 507.5. Darifenacin's absorption is rapid, with a terminal half-life of only 3 hours after single dosing and 4 to 5 hours after reaching a steady state. Clinically used darifenacin is an extended-release preparation with the following inactive ingredients: dibasic calcium phosphate anhydrous, dihydroxypropyl methylcellulose, lactose

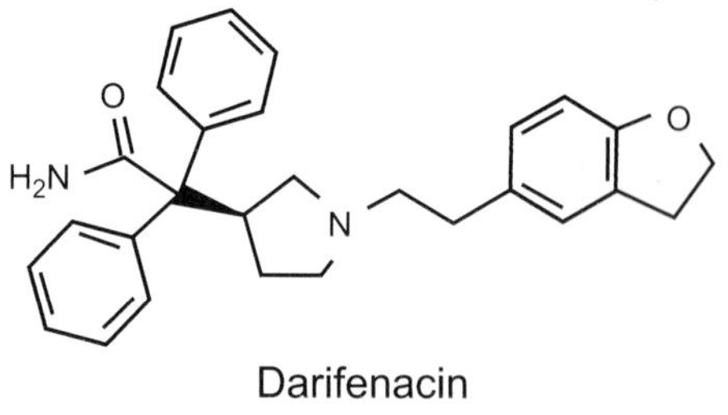

Darifenacin

Fig. 1. Chemical structure of darifenacin hydrobromide.

monohydrate, magnesium stearate, titanium dioxide, and triacetin, along with FD&C Yellow #6 Aluminum Lake. It is freely soluble in dimethyl sulfoxide and its pKa in water containing 10% methanol is 9.20. Darifenacin's polarity and molecular structure allows access to the central nervous system. In the conscious mouse, darifenacin can inhibit oxotremorine-induced tremor.

In vitro studies using human recombinant muscarinic receptors expressed in oocytes show that darifenacin has a ninefold greater affinity for the M_3 receptor compared with M_1, a 12-fold greater affinity for M_3 than M_5, and a 59-fold greater affinity for M_3 than M_2 or M_4 (Fig. 2) [25]. These in vitro data indicate that darifenacin has the greatest M_3 affinity over other muscarinic receptor subtypes compared with oxybutynin, tolterodine, solifenacin, and trospium (Table 1, see Fig. 2) [26]. In a functional assay using ^{3}H-inositol triphosphate accumulation in guinea pig tissues, darifenacin was 7.9 times more selective for detrusor than submandibular gland [26].

Pharmacokinetics

Peak plasma concentration of darifenacin in its extended release formulation after oral administration occurs at approximately 7 hours (Table 2). After daily dosing, a steady-state level of drug is achieved after 6 days. Mean bioavailability for darifenacin is 15% and 19% for 7.5- and 15-mg tablets, respectively. Food has no effect on pharmacokinetic values after a steady-state level is achieved. Darifenacin is 98% bound to plasma proteins, primarily α_1 acid glycoprotein. Its

Table 1
Muscarinic selectivity of antimuscarinics for M_1 versus M_3

Agent	M_1	M_3	Ratio
Trospium1	9.1	9.3	1.02
Tolterodine2	8.8	8.5	0.96
Oxybutynin2	8.7	8.9	1.02
Solifenacin3	7.6	8.0	1.05
Darifenacin2	8.2	9.1	1.11

volume of distribution is 163 L. These pharmacokinetic data show that darifenacin is widely distributed in the body and achieves pharmacologically active levels when administered once daily.

Metabolism of darfenacin occurs in the liver by the cytochrome P-450 enzymes CYP2D6 and CYP3A4 [27]. The metabolic enzymes differ somewhat compared with other antimuscarinics (Table 3). Initial metabolites are the product of hydroxylation and N-dealkylation. These metabolites are 3 to 10 times less potent at inhibition of bladder contractions in guinea pig and dog yet retain M_3-subtype selectivity. The hydroxylated metabolite is ninefold less potent in vivo on salivary gland secretion [28]. The half-life of darifenacin in extensive metabolizers is about 12 hours. In poor metabolizers of CYP2D6, darifenacin's half-life is 20 hours. No dosage adjustment is needed in patients who have reduced renal function. Darifenacin doses may need adjustment in patients who have hepatic dysfunction (not to exceed 7.5 mg) or are on drugs that influence the CYP2D6 and CYP3A4 enzymes. A potent CYP2D6 inhibitor is paroxetine, commonly used in the OAB

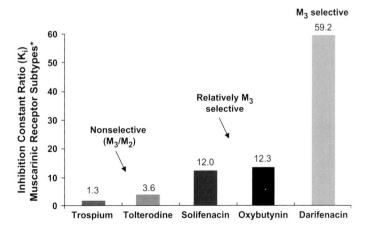

Fig. 2. M_3/M_2 receptor selectivity for darifenacin compared with other antimuscarinics.

Table 2
Pharmacokinetics for darifenacin at two approved doses

	7.5 mg qd	30 mg qd
Cmax (ng/mL)	1.98	5.25
T_{max} (h)	6.7	7.1
$T_{1/2}$ (h)	11.3	16.6

population. Darifenacin should be used with caution in combination with tricyclic antidepressants because of their metabolism by CYP2D6 and narrow therapeutic window. Conversely, in a patient in whom side effects are significant, dose reductions may be in order because that individual may be a poor metabolizer. No dose adjustments recommended for race, male versus female sex, or the elderly. Pharmacokinetic data for darifenacin are unavailable for children.

Clinical efficacy

Darifenacin has been examined in over 7000 subjects who were participants in registration or postmarketing studies. Studies were performed using 3.75 mg, 7.5 mg, 15 mg, and 30 mg for efficacy for OAB and urge incontinence. Clinical approval was sought for the 7.5- and 15-mg doses. The primary end point for registration studies was change from baseline in the median number of urge incontinent episodes at 12 weeks as noted on 7-day diaries following a 2-week washout, if appropriate, of another antimuscarinic and a 2-week placebo or drug-free run-in period. Secondary end points included change from baseline in the median number of voids and void volumes at 12 weeks. In three phase III studies, 7.5- and 15-mg doses of darifenacin reduced median urge urinary incontinence episodes per week by 68% to 71% and 73% to 84%, respectively (Fig. 3) [21,29,30]. Placebo reductions in two studies were 46% and 56%. Thus, compared with placebo, a reduction from 22% to 28% was

observed, similar to other antimuscarinic drugs. Roughly one fourth of the patients experienced greater than a 90% reduction in incontinent episodes. The high placebo rates were attributed to a "bladder training effect" because of close patient monitoring and the use of a 7-day electronic diary. Pooled analysis also demonstrated statistically significant reductions in urgency episodes, increased voided volumes, and increases in quality of life using the King's Health Questionnaire. Despite such reports, a Cochrane analysis examining several antimuscarinics including nonselective antimuscarinics and M_3-selective darifenacin concluded that statistical improvements in incontinent episodes were shown, but overall improvement of quality of life when factoring in side effects has not been adequately explored [31].

One advantage of darifenacin is flexible dosing. In one study, 59% of patients (compared with 68% of the placebo group) had few or tolerable side effects yet wanted to increase efficacy. These patients increased their dose from 7.5 mg to 15 mg [32]. This dose increase was associated with a 29.1% further reduction in urge incontinent episodes per week compared with a 12% reduction in those maintained on 7.5 mg. Dose escalation was associated with 14% fewer withdrawal rates. Perhaps most important, dose escalation was not found to increase rates of dry mouth and constipation. This observation suggests that flexible dosing with antimuscarinics may permit rapid metabolizers or those whose pharmacokinetics do not allow sufficient drug to reach the bladder to titrate doses to their optimum level.

In a study that specifically examined urgency using the concept of warning time, 72 subjects who had urgency for greater than 6 months and four or more urge episodes per day were randomized to darifenacin (30 mg) or placebo [33]. Warning time was defined as the time from first sensation to urgency, voluntary micturition, or incontinence. Darifenacin increased mean warning time by a statistically significant 4.3 minutes,

Table 3
Metabolic parameters for darifenacin

	Darifenacin	Oxybutynin	Tolterodine	Solifenacin	Trospium
Blood-brain barrier passage	Lipophilic	Lipophilic	Lipophilic	Lipophilic	Hydrophilic
Metabolism (Cytochrome P-450)	CYP2D6 CYP3A4	CYP3A4	CYP2D6	CYP3A4	Ester hydrolysis followed by conjugation
% Bioavailable active compound in urine	3%	<0.1%	<1.0% (5%–14% active metabolite)	<15.0%	60% of the bioavailable dose

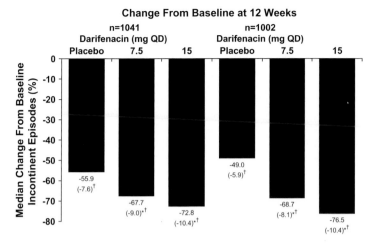

Fig. 3. Pooled analysis of phase III studies for darifenacin versus placebo on incontinent episodes.

which was thought to be clinically significant. A quality-of-life instrument, however, was not used on this small group to ascertain whether this increase in warning time was truly clinically significant. Moreover, a 30-mg dose is not approved dosing. Darifenacin treatment also statistically significantly reduced severity of urgency in clinical assessment, although this was not reflected in home diaries. This finding heightens concern about the use of home diaries as the "gold standard" for assessing urinary symptoms including incontinence. Recent unpublished data suggest that the longer the diary, the less it is accurate because subjects tend to fill out the diary the day before or the morning of their clinic appointment. The finding that darifenacin and other antimuscarinics may modulate urgency raises the possibility that acetylcholine acts on sensory mechanisms in the lower urinary tract. It has been speculated that in addition to the detrusor, muscarinic receptors on urothelium or interstitial cells are targets for antimuscarinics.

The durability of clinical response to darifenacin appears reasonable. In a 2-year open-label study of darifenacin for OAB (Haab, submitted for publication, 2006), an 84.4% reduction in the median number of incontinence episodes per week was maintained, with 66% of subjects completing this 2-year study. One caveat of open-label studies is the selection bias for inclusion of patients who tolerated the drug well or who perceived a significant enough benefit to put up with the inconvenience of the study protocol. Efficacy was redefined as per protocol, not intent

to treat, because voluntary continuation beyond the initial study could be chosen for a variety of reasons. Long-term use of antimuscarinics (persistency) can be limited by lack of efficacy or by tolerability.

Safety and tolerability

Pooled data analysis reveals that darifenacin is well tolerated and possesses typical dose-dependent side effects expected for an antimuscarinic agent. The discontinuation rate due to side effects in three phase III studies was 1.5% for a 7.5-mg dose, 5.1% for a 15-mg dose, and 2.6% for placebo. It should be appreciated, however, that discontinuation rates for trial subjects are lower than in clinical practice.

The most common side effect was dry mouth, seen in 20.2% and 35.3% on 7.5- and 15-mg doses, respectively. Constipation was the next most common side effect, seen in 14.8% and 21.3% on 7.5- and 15-mg doses, respectively. It should be noted that patients who had severe constipation, defined as less than two bowel movements per week, were excluded from these studies. The rate of constipation appears to be somewhat higher than with other antimuscarinics but did not result in a higher discontinuation rate as reported with other antimuscarinics. In the open-label 2-year extension study, 23% of subjects complained of dry mouth and 20.9% of constipation. Regardless, these side effects in a select population led to discontinuation in only

1.3% and 2.4%, respectively. In order of prevalence, other side effects included dyspepsia, abdominal pain, nausea, diarrhea, urinary tract infection, dizziness, asthenia, and dry eyes. In a comparator study with oxybutynin (5 mg three times daily), dry mouth was less common with darifenacin (13%) than with oxybutynin (36%) [34], and rates of constipation (10% for darifenacin; 8% for oxybutynin) were similar. The prevalence of dry mouth and constipation in this trial, however, was somewhat lower than in other studies of darifenacin.

One particular potential advantage of M_3-selective antimuscarinics is the lack of effect on cognition. The role of muscarinic receptors, however, is extremely complex and often based on rodent studies. Two potential side issues regarding antimuscarinics and the brain include (1) the effects on different aspects of cognition and (2) the influence on β-amyloid plaque formation. Postsynaptic M_1 receptors are required to process information between the hippocampus and the cortex. Postsynaptic M_2 receptors are required for working memory, behavioral flexibility, and learning (plasticity) [35]. Thus, it is possible that changes in memory and other aspects of cognition are affected by drugs blocking M_1/M_2 receptors. On the other hand, blockade of M_2 autoreceptors enhances cholinergic transmission and improves memory. In this case, the adverse central nervous system effects of M_2 antagonism may counteract each other. The concept that increased acetylcholine acting at M_1/M_2 receptors increases certain aspects of learning and memory forms the basis for the use of cholinesterase inhibitors such as donepezil hydrochloride in dementias and memory disturbances. Of particular interest is that estrogen modulates M_2 cholinergic function in the brain and has been thought to prevent cognitive deterioration [36]. Over 80% of subjects in registration studies for antimuscarinics are women, due to the prevalence of OAB and urge incontinence associated with the female population younger than 65 years. Whether estradiol helps prevent any cognitive changes in premenopausal women due to antimuscarinics is an intriguing conjecture.

In addition to effects on thought processing and memory, muscarinic receptors play a crucial role in processing amyloid in the brain. M_1/M_3 receptors influence cleavage of β-amyloid precursor to the nonamyloidogenic product sAPPα. In contrast, M_2 receptor activation promotes amyloidogenic sAPPβ. These facts take on heightened interest with a report that patients who have Parkinson's disease and are on anticholinergics (primarily tricyclic antidepressants) were found to have increased plaques and neurofibrillary tangles in autopsied brains [37]. Whether use of antimuscarinics promotes or prevents plaque in humans who have early dementias or are predisposed to Alzheimer's disease is unknown.

What is known is that antimuscarinics can influence cognition. Tertiary amines such as oxybutynin, propantheline, hyoscyamine, and scopolamine readily access the cerebrospinal fluid (see Table 3). The quaternary amine trospium hydrochloride does not. Tolterodine, being somewhat more polar, does not achieve high cerebrospinal fluid levels at recommended doses. Oxybutynin and tolterodine have been shown to affect cognition and sleep in humans and animals [38–41]. In an assessment of cognitive function in the elderly, darifenacin did not affect memory scanning, speed of choice, reaction time, or word-recognition sensitivity [42]. The prohibition on the simultaneous use of drugs such as donepezil and antimuscarinics is logical but has not been specifically studied. Whether an M_3-selective antimuscarinic drug such as darifenacin can be safely used in patients who have dementias or are on donepezil is an intriguing possibility. Because many patients who have dementias suffer from urinary incontinence due to detrusor overactivity, an antimuscarinic combined with prompted voiding might be advantageous. In one small study, seven of eight patients who had Alzheimer's disease and were undergoing urodynamics exhibited detrusor overactivity, indicating that incontinence is not merely due to lack of attention [43]. Administration of donepezil was beneficial for incontinence. Whether this benefit was due to cholinergic activity on micturition pathways or the bladder or due to improved cognition was not determined, but there are hints that combined drug approaches might possess therapeutic benefit. Although one group of investigators suggested that combining an antimuscarinic and acetylcholinesterase inhibitor is safe [44], another group recently found that antimuscarinics worsen mental status and behavior in patients who have Alzheimer's disease [45].

One purported advantage of M_3-selective antagonists is the lack of effect on the heart. In a comparator trial of darifenacin and oxybutynin, no differences in resting heart rate or heart rate variability between these two drugs was observed [22]. Penile erection, another vascular process, could theoretically be adversely affected by antimuscarinics. Acetylcholine facilitates endothelial-mediated relaxation of the corpus cavernosum. The human penis expresses M_1, M_2, M_3, and M_4 receptor RNA [46]. Of these receptors, the M_2 and M_4 subtypes are thought to modulate corpus cavernosum tone [46]. Although sexual dysfunction including erectile dysfunction has not been specifically studied with darifenacin, an Italian population-based study found that anticholinergic drugs were associated with risk for erectile dysfunction (odds ratio: 12.8; 95% confidence interval: 2.17–60.1) [47]. Cholinergic mechanisms also influence central mechanisms involved in ejaculatory function in animals; however, reports of changes in emission and ejaculation in humans have not been investigated.

Summary

Darifenacin is an effective drug for the treatment of OAB and is tolerated by patients. Darifenacin's M_3 selectivity is unique among antimuscarinics. This M_3 selectivity could confer advantages in patients who have cardiovascular side effects (tachycardia), impaired cognition, complaints of dizziness, or sleep disturbances. In some studies, darifenacin caused less dry mouth than oxybutynin. Rates of constipation, although significant, are tolerated and rarely a cause for discontinuation in clinical trials.

References

[1] Croom KF, Keating GM. Darifenacin in the treatment of overactive bladder. Drugs Aging 2004; 21(13):885–92.

[2] Andersson KE, Arner A. Urinary bladder contraction and relaxation: physiology and pathophysiology. Physol Rev 2004;84(3):935–86.

[3] Andersson KE, Wein AJ. Pharmacology of the lower urinary tract: basis for current and future treatments of urinary incontinence. Pharmacol Rev 2004; 56(4):581–631.

[4] Chess-Williams R, Chapple CR, Yamanishi T, et al. The minor population of M3-receptors mediate contraction of human detrusor muscle in vitro. J Auton Pharmacol 2001;21(5–6):243–8.

[5] Boselli C, Govoni S, Vicini D, et al. Presence and passage dependent loss of biochemical M3 muscarinic receptor function in human detrusor cultured smooth muscle cells. J Urol 2002;168(6):2672–6.

[6] Fetscher C, Fleichman M, Schmidt M, et al. M(3) muscarinic receptors mediate contraction of human urinary bladder. Br J Pharmacol 2002;136(5):641–3.

[7] Miyamae K, Yoshida M, Murakami S, et al. Pharmacologic effects of darifenacin on human

isolated urinary bladder. Pharmacology 2003; 69(4):205–11.

[8] Schneider T, Fetscher C, Kresge S, et al. Signal transduction underlying carbachol-induced contraction of human urinary bladder. J Pharmacol Exp Ther 2004;309(3):1148–53.

[9] Mansfield KJ, Mitchelson FJ, Moore KH, et al. Muscarinic receptor subtypes in the human colon: lack of evidence for atypical subtypes. Eur J Pharmacol 2003;482(1–3):101–9.

[10] Matsui M, Motomura D, Karasawa H, et al. Multiple functional defects in peripheral autonomic organs in mice lacking muscarinic acetylcholine receptor gene for the M3 subtype. Proc Natl Acad Sci U S A 2000;97(17):9579–84.

[11] Stengel PW, Yamada M, Wess J, et al. M(3)-receptor knockout mice: muscarinic receptor function in atria, stomach fundus, urinary bladder, and trachea. Am J Physiol Regul Integr Comp Physiol 2002; 282(5):R1443–9.

[12] Lapides J, Hodgson NB, Boyd RE. Effect of adrenolytic, adrenergic, anticholinergic, cholinergic and antihistaminic drugs on micturition. Surg Forum 1957; 8:650–3.

[13] Pontari MA, Braverman AS, Ruggieri MR Sr. The M2 muscarinic receptor mediates in vitro bladder contractions from patients with neurogenic bladder dysfunction. Am J Physiol 2004;286(5):R874–80.

[14] Braverman AS, Ruggieri MR Sr. Hypertrophy changes the muscarinic receptor subtype mediating bladder contraction from M3 to M2. Am J Physiol Regul Integr Comp Physiol 2003;285(3):R701–8.

[15] Tong YC, Cheng JT. Alteration of M(3) subtype muscarinic receptors in the diabetic rat urinary bladder. Pharmacology 2002;64(3):148–51.

[16] Ishizuka O, Gu BJ, Yang ZX, et al. Functional role of central muscarinic receptors for micturition in normal conscious rats. J Urol 2002;168(5):2258–62.

[17] Modiri AR, Alberts P, Gillberg PG. Effect of muscarinic antagonists on micturition pressure measured by cystometry in normal, conscious rats. Urology 2002;59(6):963–8.

[18] Mansfield KJ, Liu L, Mitchelson FJ, et al. Muscarinic receptor subtypes in human bladder detrusor and mucosa, studied by radioligand binding and quantitative competitive RT-PCR: changes in ageing. Br J Pharmacol 2005;144(8):1089–99.

[19] Culp DJ, Luo W, Richardson LA, et al. Both M1 and M3 receptors regulate exocrine secretion by mucinous acini. Am J Physiol 1996;271:C1963–72.

[20] Gillberg PG, Sundquist S, Nilvebrant L. Comparison of the in vitro and in vivo profiles of tolterodine with those of subtype-selective muscarinic receptor antagonists. Eur J Pharmacol 1998;349(2): 285–92.

[21] Chapple CR, Abrams P. Comparison of darefinacin and oxybutynin in patients with overactive bladder: assessment of ambulatory urodynamics and impact on salivary flow. Eur Urol 2005;48(1):102–9.

[22] Brodde OE, Bruck H, Leineweber K, et al. Presence, distribution and physiologic function of adrenergic and muscarinic receptor subtypes in the human heart. Basic Res Cardiol 2001;96(6):528–38.

[23] Serra DB, Affrime MB, Bedigian MP, et al. QT and QTc interval with standard and supratherapeutic doses of darifenacin, a muscarinic M3 selective receptor antagonist for the treatment of overactive bladder. J Clin Pharmacol 2005;45(9):1038–47.

[24] Wang Z, Shi H, Wang H. Functional M3 muscarinic acetylcholine receptors in mammalian hearts. Br J Pharmacol 2004;142(3):395–408.

[25] Smith CM, Wallis RM. Characterization of [3H]-darifenacin as a novel radioligand for the study of muscarinic M3 receptors. J Recept Signal Transduct Res 1997;17(1–3):177–84.

[26] Nelson CP, Gupta P, Napier CM, et al. Functional selectivity of muscarinic receptor antagonists for inhibition of M3-mediated phosphoinositide responses in guinea pig urinary bladder and submandibular salivary gland. J Pharmacol Exp Ther 2004;310(3):1255–65.

[27] Kerbusch T, Wahlby U, Milligan PA, et al. Population pharmacokinetic modelling of darifenacin and its hydroxylated metabolite using pooled data, incorporating saturable first-pass metabolism, CYP2D6 genotype and formulation-dependent bioavailability. Br J Clin Phamracol 2003;56(6):639–52.

[28] Kerbusch T, Milligan PA, Karlsson MO. Assessment of the relative in vivo potency of the hydroxylated metabolite of darifenacin in its ability to decrease salivary flow using pooled population pharmacokinetic-pharmacodynamic data. Br J Clin Pharmacol 2004;57(2):170–80.

[29] Haab F. Darifenacin in the treatment of overactive bladder. Drugs Today 2005;41(7):441–52.

[30] Chapple CR. Darifenacin: a novel M3 muscarinic selective receptor antagonist for the treatment of overactive bladder. Expert Opin Investig Drugs 2004;13(11):1493–500.

[31] Hay-Smith J, Herbison O, Ellis G, et al. Anticholinergic drugs versus placebo for overactive bladder syndrome in adults. Cochrane Database Syst Rev 2005;4:CD003781.

[32] Steers WJ, Corcos J, Foote J, et al. An investigation of dose titration with darifenacin, an M3-selective receptor antagonist. BJU Int 2005;95(4):580–6.

[33] Cardozo L, Dixon A. Increased warning time with darifenacin: a new concept in the management of urinary urgency. J Urol 2005;173(4):1214–8.

[34] Zinner N, Tuttle J, Marks L. Efficacy and tolerability of darifenacin, a muscarinic M3 selective receptor antagonist (M3 SRA), compared with oxybutynin in the treatment of patients with overactive bladder. World J Urol 2005;23(4):248–52.

[35] Seeger T, Fedorova I, Zheng F, et al. M2 muscarinic acetylcholine receptor knock-out mice show deficits in behavioral flexibility, working memory, and hippocampal plasticity. J Neurosci 2004;24(45):10117–27.

[36] Daniel JM, Hulst JL, Lee CD. Role of hippocampal M2 muscarinic receptors in the estrogen-induced enhancement of working memory. Neuroscience 2005;132:57–64.

[37] Perry EK, Kilford L, Lees AJ, et al. Increased Alzheimer pathology in Parkinson's disease related to antimuscarinic drugs. Ann Neurol 2003;54:235–8.

[38] Sugiyama T, Park YC, Kurita T. Oxybutynin disrupts learning and memory in the rat passive avoidance response. Urol Res 1999;27:393–5.

[39] Womack KB, Heilman KM. Tolterodine and memory: dry but forgetful. Arch Neurol 2003;60(5):771–3.

[40] Todorova A, Vonderheid-Guth B, Dimpfel W. Effects of tolterodine, trospium chloride, and oxybutynin on the central nervous system. J Clin Phamracol 2001;41(6):636–44.

[41] Diefenbach K, Arold G, Wollny A, et al. Effects on sleep of anticholinergics used for overactive bladder treatment in healthy volunteers aged > 50 years. Br J Urol 2003;95(3):346.

[42] Lipton RB, Kolodner K, Wesnes K. Assessment of cognitive function of the elderly population: effects of darifenacin. J Urol 2005;173(2):493–8.

[43] Sakakibara R, Uchiyama T, Yoshiyama M, et al. Preliminary communication: urodynamic assessment of donepezil hydrochloride in patients with Alzheimer's disease. Neurourol Urodynam 2005;24(3):273–5.

[44] Siegler EL, Reidenberg M. Treatment of urinary incontinence with anticholinergics in patients taking cholinesterase inhibitors for dementias. Clin Pharmacol Ther 2004;75(5):484–8.

[45] Jewart RD, Green J, Lu CJ, et al. Cognitive, behavioral and physiological changes in Alzheimer disease patients as a function of incontinence medications. Amer J Geriat Psych 2005;13(4):324–8.

[46] Traish A, Kim NN, Huang YH, et al. Expression of functional muscarinic acetylcholine receptor subtypes in human corpus cavernosum and in cultured smooth muscle cells. Receptor 1995;5(3):159–76.

[47] Ricci E, Parazzini F, Mirone V, et al. Current drug use as risk factor for erectile dysfunction: results from an Italian epidemiological study. Inter J Impotence Res 2003;15(3):221–4.

ELSEVIER
SAUNDERS

Urol Clin N Am 33 (2006) 483–490

UROLOGIC
CLINICS
of North America

Solifenacin

Karl J. Kreder, MD

Department of Urology, University of Iowa, 200 Hawkins Drive, 3 RCP, Iowa City, IA 52242-1089, USA

Overactive bladder syndrome (OAB) is defined by the International Continence Society as being comprised of the symptoms of urgency with or without urge incontinence and is usually accompanied by frequency and nocturia [1]. OAB is a common condition, estimated to affect between 16% and 22% of American adults, with even higher rates in the elderly [2,3]. The treatment options for OAB include behavioral, pharmacologic, and surgical therapy. Because the newer agents are long-acting, once-a-day dosing is possible. The newer agents also have better side effect profiles compared with short-acting antimuscarinic drugs. Solifenacin succinate is a new once-daily antimuscarinic agent that is discussed in this article.

Chemistry

Solifenacin is a tertiary amine with demonstrated antimuscarinic properties. The chemical formula and the chemical structure of solifenacin are illustrated in Fig. 1. Solifenacin has a molecular weight of 480.55.

Pharmacokinetics

T_{max} and $T_{1/2}$

In a multidosing study (5, 10, 20, and 30 mg) conducted in young men, the time to maximal plasma concentration (T_{max}) for solifenacin ranged from 2.9 hours for the 20-mg dose to 5.8 hours for the 5-mg dose. The terminal elimination half-life ($T_{1/2}$) was 45 hours and 64 hours, respectively [4]. The steady state of solifenacin was reached after 10 days of therapy (Figs. 2 and 3).

E-mail address: karl-kreder@uiowa.edu

Metabolism and elimination

Solifenacin is extensively metabolized in the liver by the cytochrome P (CYP)3A4 enzyme pathway. In a study of healthy volunteers, only 15% of ^{14}C-radiolabeled solifenacin was recovered in the urine as intact solifenacin, and 69.2% of the radioactive solifenacin was recovered in the urine as metabolites of solifenacin and 22.5% was recovered in the feces [5].

Special considerations

In one study, volunteers aged 65 to 80 years had a 16% and 20% higher average urinary concentration (AUC) and C_{max}, respectively, than younger (18–55 years) volunteers [6]. In clinical trials, however, similar safety and efficacy were demonstrated in patients older and younger than 65 years [7].

No dose adjustments are necessary for sex, and not enough data are available to make any comment about the pharmacokinetics in different races. In patients who have severe renal impairment, there is a 2.1-fold increase in the AUC and a 1.6 increase in the $T_{1/2}$ [8]. In patients who have moderate hepatic impairment, there is a twofold increase in the $T_{1/2}$ and a 35% increase in the AUC.

Mechanism of action

There are five subtypes of muscarinic receptors in the human body (M_1–M_5). The M_2 and M_3 receptors play a role in bladder function [9–11]. Approximately 80% of the muscarinic receptors in the bladder are of the M_2 subtype and 20% are of the M_3 subtype. Although the M_3 receptor is more prevalent than the M_2 receptor in the healthy human bladder, M_3 is the receptor

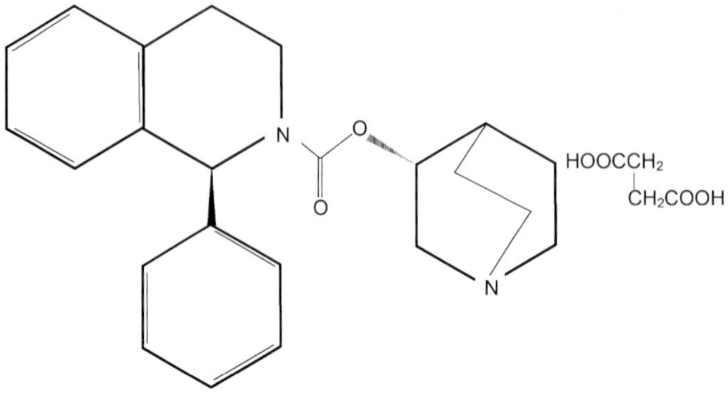

Fig. 1. Structural formula of solifenacin succinate.

primarily responsible for bladder contraction. Stimulation of the M_3 receptor causes a direct contraction of the detrusor smooth muscle by way of phosphoinositide hydrolysis. Although the functional role of the M_2 receptor has not been completely clarified, it appears that activation of the M_2 receptor may oppose the sympathetically mediated smooth muscle relaxation, thereby causing bladder contraction [12]. The M_2 receptor may play a more important role in bladder contraction than the M_3 receptor in disease states such as neurogenic bladder dysfunction [9]. The M_3 receptor is also present in the salivary glands and intestine and, therefore, blockade of the M_3 receptor in the bladder results in blockade of M_3 receptors in these organs. M_3 receptor binding in the intestine and salivary glands leads to the most common side effects of this agent and of this class of agents: xerostomia (dry mouth) and constipation.

In animal models (guinea pig and mouse), Ikeda and colleagues [5] compared the binding characteristics of solifenacin and oxybutynin. In radioactive ligand-binding assays, pKi values of solifenacin for M_1, M_2, and M_3 receptors were 7.6, 6.9, and 8.0, respectively. For oxybutynin, these values were 8.6, 7.7, and 8.9, respectively. To study the tissue selectivity between bladder and the salivary gland, guinea pig detrusor and mouse submandibular gland cells were stimulated with carbochol and intracellular calcium measured. Calcium mobilization of the detrusor cells was inhibited equipotentially by solifenacin (pKi = 8.4) and by oxybutynin (pKi = 8.6), but salivary gland cells were antagonized less potently (pKb = 7.4) by solifenacin than they were by oxybutynin

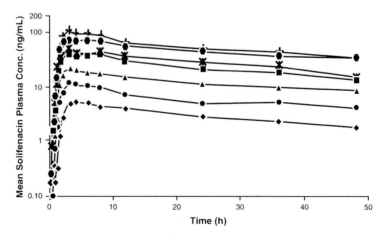

Fig. 2. Mean plasma concentration versus time profiles obtained after oral administration of single 5-mg to 100-mg doses of solifenacin. (*From* Smulders RA, Krauwinkel WJ, Swart PJ, et al. Pharmakokinetics and safety of solifenacin succinate in healthy young men. J Clin Pharmacol 2004;44:1027; with permission.)

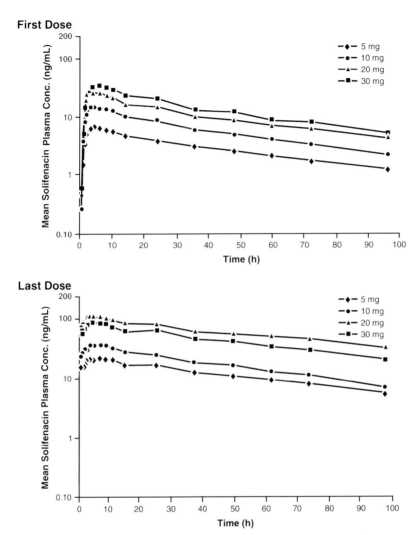

Fig. 3. Mean plasma concentration versus time profiles obtained after the first and last doses of solifenacin in the multi-dose study. (*From* Smulders RA, Krauwinkel WJ, Swart PJ, et al. Pharmakokinetics and safety of solifenacin succinate in healthy young men. J Clin Pharmacol 2004;44:1027; with permission.)

(pKb = 8.8), even though both responses are mediated by the M_3 receptor. The investigators concluded that the M_3 receptor antagonism by solifenacin may be bladder selective.

In a second study, Ohtake and colleagues [13] evaluated the bladder selectivity profile of solifenacin over the salivary gland in a single animal species, the male Wistar rat. They compared the results obtained for solifenacin to those for tolterodine, oxybutynin, darifenacin, and atropine. These investigators reported that all of the antimuscarinic agents studied in their animal model inhibited carbachol-induced increase of intracellular calcium levels in vitro in bladder smooth muscle and salivary gland cells in a dose-dependent manner. Solifenacin and tolterodine demonstrated selectivity for bladder smooth muscle cells over salivary gland cells, whereas oxybutynin, darifenacin, and atropine did not. The same investigators reported that in anesthetized Wistar rats, solifenacin and tolterodine dose-dependently inhibited carbochol-induced intravesical pressure elevation and salivary secretion, and exhibited functional selectivity for urinary bladder over the salivary gland. In contrast, oxybutynin, darifenacin, and atropine did not. The investigators concluded that in this study, the estimated rank order for urinary bladder selectivity was solifenacin greater than tolterodine greater than oxybutynin equal to darifenacin equal to atropine.

Kobayashi and colleagues [14] examined the in vitro effects of solifenacin, tolterodine, oxybutynin, and darifenacin in a nonhuman primate model (monkey) using bladder smooth muscle cells and some mandibular gland cells. They reported pKi ratios of submandibular gland/bladder cells of 2.1 for solifenacin, 0.65 for tolterodine, 0.51 for oxybutynin, and 0.46 for darifenacin. These investigators concluded that in this model, solifenacin demonstrated greater bladder selectivity than tolterodine, oxybutynin, or darifenacin.

Drug–drug interactions

Solifenacin is primarily metabolized in the liver in the CYP3A4 pathway. Inducers or inhibitors of CYP3A4 may alter solifenacin pharmacokinetics.

Michel and colleagues [15] studied the interaction of solifenacin and warfarin in 12 healthy men (mean age 24.9 years) who had a mean body weight of 75.3 kg and in 12 male and 12 female subjects (mean age 28.7 years) who had a mean body weight of 72 kg. They concluded that administration of 10 mg of solifenacin once daily with a single 25-mg dose of warfarin or a 0.25-mg

loading dose of digoxin followed by 1.25 mg was well tolerated.

Uchida and colleagues [16] examined the effect of food ingestion on the pharmacokinetic profile of solifenacin and in a randomized, crossover study of 24 healthy men (aged 18–45 years, body weight 60–100 kg, mean body mass index ≤ 30). A single 10-mg dose was administered to the first group in the fasting state during period 1 and in the fed state during period 2. The same dose was administered to the second group in the fed state during period 1 and the fasting state during period 2. The measured parameters included C_{max}, AUC, $T_{1/2max}$, and T_{max}. The investigators concluded that the pharmacokinetic of oral solifenacin was not affected by food ingestion.

Clinical trials

Chapple and colleagues [7] reported on a multi-center randomized trial that involved 1281 patients who had OAB symptoms, in which 1077 were treated. After placebo run-in, patients were randomized in equal numbers to 12 weeks of double-blind treatment with tolterodine (2 mg twice daily), to placebo, or to solifenacin (5 or 10 mg once daily). Patients were evaluated with voiding dairies at baseline, 4 weeks, and 12 weeks. The efficacy variables included change from baseline in the mean number of episodes of urgency,

Table 1
Number (%) of patients discontinuing treatment before study completion and the treatment-related major anticholinergic side effects

| Characteristic | Placebo (n = 267) | Solifenacin (once daily) | | Tolterodine (twice daily) | Total (N = 1077) |
		5 mg (n = 279)	10 mg (n = 268)	2 mg (n = 263)	
Discontinuing					
Adverse event	10 (3.7)	9 (3.2)	7 (2.6)	5 (1.9)	31 (2.9)
Consent withdrawal	10 (3.7)	11 (3.9)	7 (2.6)	8 (3.0)	36 (3.3)
Lost to follow-up	2 (0.7)	1 (0.4)	2 (0.7)	6 (2.3)	11 (1.0)
Protocol violation	5 (1.9)	4 (1.4)	0	3 (1.1)	12 (1.1)
Insufficient response	2 (0.7)	2 (0.7)	1 (0.4)	3 (1.1)	8 (0.7)
Patient died	0	0	1 (0.4)	1 (0.4)	2 (0.2)
Other	3 (1.1)	1 (0.4)	1 (0.4)	0	5 (0.5)
Total	32 (12.0)	28 (10.0)	19 (7.1)	26 (9.9)	105 (9.7)
Major side effects					
Dry mouth	13 (4.9)	39 (14.0)	57 (21.3)	49 (18.6)	
Constipation	5 (1.9)	20 (7.2)	21 (7.8)	7 (2.6)	
Blurred vision	7 (2.6)	10 (3.6)	15 (5.6)	4 (1.5)	

Data from Chapple CR, Rechberger T, Al-Shukri S, et al, on behalf of the YM-905 Study Group. Randomized, double-blind placebo- and tolterodine-controlled trial of the once-daily antimuscarinic agent solifenacin in patients with symptomatic overactive bladder. BJU Int 2004;93(3):309.

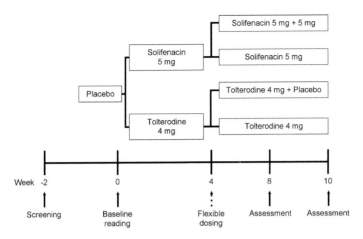

Fig. 4. STAR trial study design. (*From* Chapple CR, Martinez-Garcia R, Selvaggi L, et al. A comparison of the efficacy and tolerability of solifenacin succinate and extended release tolterodine at treating overactive bladder syndrome: results of the STAR trial. Eur Urol 2005;48(3):465; with permission. © 2005, European Association of Urology.)

incontinence, and urgent continence. Patients treated with solifenacin demonstrated a significant decrease from baseline and the number of urgency episodes per 24 hours compared with placebo (placebo, 33%; 5-mg solifenacin, 52%; 10-mg solifenacin, 55%; $P < 0.001$).

Solifenacin produced statistically significant reductions in all incontinent episodes versus placebo: 5-mg solifenacin, -1.42 episodes per day, $P = 0.008$; 10-mg solifenacin, -1.45 episodes per day, $P = 0.0038$). Table 1 demonstrates the side effects reported in this trial.

A subsequent flexible dosing trial of solifenacin (Solifenacin and Tolterodine as an Active comparator in a Randomized (STAR) trial) was reported by Chapple and colleagues [17]. In this study, the primary end point was powered for noninferiority, and solifenacin in a 5-mg or 10-mg dose was compared with tolterodine in a formula gram dose. Four weeks into the trial, patients could escalate their dose of solifenacin from 5 mg to 10 mg after consultation with their physician. Patients in the tolterodine trial (4 mg) were escalated to 4 mg tolterodine plus 4 mg placebo. The design of this trail is illustrated in Fig. 4. For the primary end point of reduction of micturition frequency, solifenacin was found to be as effective as tolterodine ($P = 0.004$, noninferiority) (Fig. 5). Solifenacin demonstrated improvement in secondary outcome measures including urge incontinence ($P = 0.001$), overall incontinence ($P = 0.006$), and urgency ($P = 0.035$) compared with the patients who were treated with 4 mg of extended-release tolterodine (Table 2). Fifty-nine

percent of the patients treated with solifenacin were dry at the end of this trial compared with 49% who were treated with tolterodine ($P = 0.006$), although the numbers were pooled and not specifically reported for the solifenacin 5-mg dose versus the 10-mg dose. The overall discontinuation rates were 5.9% for solifenacin and 7.3% for extended-release tolterodine.

Cardozo and colleagues [18] reported on 1091 enrolled and 907 treated patients in a multinational 12-week randomized, placebo-controlled trial comparing placebo to 5- and 10-mg doses of solifenacin. The primary efficacy variable was the change from baseline in the mean number of micturitions per 24 hours. Secondary efficacy variables included the change from baseline to the end of the study in the mean number of urgency episodes per 24 hours, nocturia, urge continence, all incontinence, and voided volume per micturition. All efficacy variables were based on a 3-day voiding dairy. Solifenacin 5- and 10-mg doses

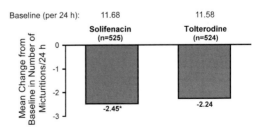

Fig. 5. Baseline to end point change in OAB symptoms from the STAR trial.

Table 2
Secondary end points from the STAR trial

End point	Solifenacin Mean change from baseline	Tolterodine Mean change from baseline	P Solifenacin versus Tolterodine
Incontinence episodes/24 h	−1.60	−1.11	0.006
Urge incontinence episodes/24 h	−1.42	−0.83	0.001
Pads used/24 h	−1.72	−1.19	0.002
Urgency episodes/24 h	−2.85	−2.42	0.035
Volume voided/micturition (mL)	+37.95	+31.00	0.010

demonstrated a statistically significant reduction in the mean number of micturitions per 24 hours compared with placebo: placebo, −1.59 micturitions per day; 5-mg solifenacin, −2.37 micturitions per day; and 10-mg solifenacin, −2.81 micturitions per day. Fig. 5 summarizes primary and secondary outcomes in this trial.

Dry mouth was reported by 2.3% of patients receiving placebo, 7.7% of patients receiving 5 mg of solifenacin, and 23.1% of patients receiving 10 mg of solifenacin. The constipation rates were placebo, 2%; 5-mg solifenacin, 3.7%; and 10-mg solifenacin, 9.1%. Blurry vision was no more common on activate agent than placebo.

Haab and colleagues [19] reported on a trial that enrolled patients on 40 weeks of open-label solifenacin following completion of the 12-week trials previously described. Of 1802 patients who completed the 12-week randomized trials and were eligible for enrollment in the extension trial, 1637 (91%) elected to enter the extension trial.

All patients were started on solifenacin, 5 mg, and dosing adjustment was allowed up or down at 16-, 20-, and 40-week time points (Fig. 6). Efficacy variables were based on the results of a 3-day voiding diary that was completed before baseline, at each follow-up visit, and at the end of the study. Efficacy variables included the change from baseline per day and the mean number of urgency episodes, micturitions, all incontinent episodes, urgent continent episodes, nocturia episodes, and voided volume per micturition. Eighty-one percent of the patients who enrolled in the trial completed the 40-week extension. Efficacy analysis of all solifenacin-treated patients demonstrated that the mean number of incontinent episodes decreased by 66%. The mean number of micturitions per 24 hours decreased by 23%, the

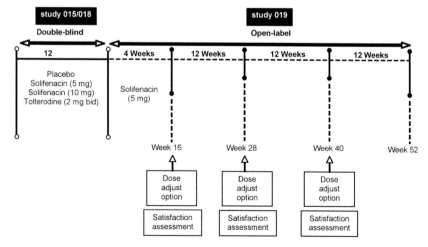

Fig. 6. Open-label extension study design. (*From* Haab F, Cardozo L, Chapple C, et al, for the Solifenacin Study Group. Long-term open-label solifenacin treatment associated with persistence with therapy in patients with overactive bladder syndrome. Eur Urol 2005;47:378; with permission. © 2005, European Association of Urology.)

Table 3
Number (%) of patients who had expected solifenacin treatment-emergent anticholinergic side effects by severity for all patients

	Patients on solifenacin 5 mg at AE report (n = 1633)	Patients on solifenacin 10 mg at AE report (n = 1114)	All patients on solifenacin (n = 1633)
Dry mouth			
Mild	132 (8.1)	122 (11.0)	235 (14.4)
Moderate	28 (1.7)	56 (5.0)	82 (5.0)
Severe	6 (0.4)	16 (1.4)	22 (1.3)
Constipation			
Mild	56 (3.4)	49 (4.4)	96 (5.9)
Moderate	19 (1.2)	27 (2.4)	44 (2.7)
Severe	5 (0.3)	12 (1.1)	17 (1.0)
Blurred vision			
Mild	49 (3.0)	39 (3.5)	85 (5.2)
Moderate	16 (1.0)	9 (0.8)	25 (1.5)
Severe	2 (0.1)	1 (0.1)	3 (0.2)

Adverse events during solifenacin treatment were recorded during 52 weeks of treatment for all patients in the extension study.

Abbreviation: AE, adverse event.

Data from Haab F, Cardozo L, Chapple C, et al, for the Solifenacin Study Group. Long-term open-label solifenacin treatment associated with persistence with therapy in patients with overactive bladder syndrome. Eur Urol 2005;47(3):380.

mean number of urgency episodes per 24 hours decreased by 63%, and nocturic episodes per 24 hours decreased by 32%. The voided volume per micturition increased by 31%, and nocturia decreased by 50%. Urgent incontinent episodes in this trial decreased by a median 100%. Sixty percent of the patients who had urge incontinence at baseline were dry after 52 weeks of solifenacin therapy and 74% of patients rated the efficacy of solifenacin as satisfactory. Reported side effects included dry mouth, constipation, and blurry vision (Table 3).

Kelleher and colleagues [20] analyzed data on quality-of-life variables from two 12-week multinational, multicentered, double-blind, randomized trials in a 40-week open-label extension of these 12-week trials. These trials enrolled men and women who were randomized to placebo or to solifenacin in 5-mg or 10-mg doses.

King's Health Questionnaire is a validated quality-of-life questionnaire with a total of 32 questions intended to identify individual bladder problems [20]. It was administered at the start of the blinded portion of the 12-week trial and at 4 and 12 weeks after the start of therapy. A total of 1890 patients provided quality-of-life data from the 12-week trial. Statistically significant differences at both solifenacin doses versus placebo were observed for all domains except personal relationships after the 12-week randomized trials.

For solifenacin 5- and 10-mg doses, data from the 40-week extension trial demonstrated improvement in all quality-of-life domains. From the start of open-label extension (from the end of the 12-week randomized trial to the end of the extension trial), the improvement was 17% for general health perception and 35% to 48% improvement for all other domains.

Summary

Solifenacin at doses of 5 mg/d and 10 mg/d is an effective and well-tolerated treatment option for patients who have OAB. Solifenacin increases functional bladder capacity and decreases urgency, frequency, and incontinence. In pharmacokinetic studies, solifenacin demonstrated selectivity for the bladder over the salivary glands; thus, it is likely that the bladder selectivity of this agent is responsible for the low incidence of dry mouth and constipation reported in the clinical trials.

References

[1] Abrams P, Cardozo L, Fall M, et al. The standardisation of terminology in lower urinary tract function: report from the Standardisation Sub-committee of the International Continence Society. Urology 2003;61(1):37–49.

[2] Stewart W, Herzog R, Wein A. Prevalence and impact of overactive bladder in the US: results from the NOBLE program. Neurourol Urodynam 2001; 20:406–8.

[3] Versi E. Screening initiative confirms widespread prevalence of overactive bladder in American adults. Int Urogynecol J 2001;12:S13.

[4] Smulders RA, Krauwinkel WJ, Swart PJ, et al. Pharmakokinetics and safety of solifenacin succinate in healthy young men. J Clin Pharmacol 2004;44(9): 1023–33.

[5] Ikeda K, Kobayashi S, Suzuki M, et al. M_3 receptor antagonism by the novel antimuscarinic agent solifenacin in the urinary bladder and salivary gland. Arch Pharmacol 2002;366(2):97–103.

[6] Krauwinkel WJ, Smulders RA, Mulder H, et al. Effect of age on the pgarmacokinetics of solifenacin in men and women. Int J Pharmacol Ther 2005;43(5):227–38.

[7] Chapple CR, Rechberger T, Al-Shukri S, et al, on behalf of the YM-905 Study Group. Randomized, double-blind placebo- and tolterodine-controlled trial of the once-daily antimuscarinic agent solifenacin in patients with symptomatic overactive bladder. BJU Int 2004;93(3):303–10.

[8] Astellas Pharma, US, Inc. and the GlaxoSmithKline Group of Companies. Prescribing information: VESIcare®. Available at: www.vesicare.com/pdf/ vesicare_prescribing_info.pdf.

[9] Andersson K-E, Wein AJ. Pharmacology of the lower urinary tract: basis for current and future treatments of urinary incontinence. Pharmacol Rev 2004;56(4):581–631.

[10] Yamaguchi O, Shishido K, Tamura K, et al. Evaluation of mRNAs encoding muscarinic receptor subtypes in human detrusor muscle. J Urol 1996;156(3): 1208–13.

[11] Sigala S, Mirabella G, Peroni A, et al. Differential gene expresion of cholonergic muscarinic receptor subtypes in male and female normal human urinary bladder. Urology 2002;60(4):719–25.

[12] Nakamura T, Kimura J, Yamaguchi O. Muscarinic M2 receptors inhibit Ca^{2+}-activated K+ channels in rat bladder smooth muscle. Int J Urol 2002;9(12): 689–96.

[13] Ohtake A, Ukai M, Hatanaka T, et al. In vitro and in vivo tissue selectivity profile of solifenacin succinate (YM905) for urinary bladder over salivary gland in rats. Eur J Pharmacol 2004;492(2–3): 243–50.

[14] Kobayashi S, Ikeda K, Miyata K. Comparison of in vitro selectivity profiles of solifenacin succinate (YM905) and current antimuscarinic drugs in bladder and salivary glands: a Ca^{2+} mobilization study in monkey cells. Life Sci 2004;74(7):843–53.

[15] Michel MC, Minematsu T, Hashimoto T, et al. In vitro studies on the potential of solifenacin for drug-drug interactions: plasma protein binding and MDR1 transport [abstract]. Br J Clin Pharmacol 2005;59(5):647.

[16] Uchida T, Krauwinkel WJ, Mulder H, et al. Food does not affect the pharmacokinetics of solifenacin, a new muscarinic receptor antagonist: results of a randomized crossover trial. Br J Clin Pharmacol 2004;58(1):4–7.

[17] Chapple CR, Martinez-Garcia R, Selvaggi L, et al. A comparison of the efficacy and tolerability of solifenacin succinate and extended release tolterodine at treating overactive bladder syndrome: results of the STAR trial. Eur Urol 2005;48(3): 464–70.

[18] Cardozo L, Lisec M, Millard R, et al. Randomized, double-blind placebo controlled trial of the once daily antimuscarinic agent solifenacin succinate in patients with overactive bladder. J Urol 2004; 172(5):1919–24.

[19] Haab F, Cardozo L, Chapple C, et al, for the Solifenacin Study Group. Long-term open-label solifenacin treatment associated with persistence with therapy in patients with overactive bladder syndrome. Eur Urol 2005;47(3):376–84.

[20] Kelleher CJ, Cardozo L, Chapple CR, et al. Improved quality of life in patients with overactive bladder symptoms treated with solifenacin. BJU Int 2005;95(1):81–5.

ELSEVIER
SAUNDERS

Urol Clin N Am 33 (2006) 491–501

UROLOGIC
CLINICS
of North America

Sacral Nerve Stimulation for the Overactive Bladder

Wendy W. Leng, MD*, Shelby N. Morrisroe, MD

*Department of Urology, University of Pittsburgh School of Medicine,
3471 Fifth Avenue, Suite 700, Pittsburgh, PA 15213, USA*

The refractory overactive bladder (OAB) represents one of the most challenging problems in general urology practice. Although rarely a life-threatening condition, the impact on individual quality of life in the physical and psychosocial domains is undeniable [1]. Furthermore, recent epidemiologic surveys confirm our clinical sense that prevalence of the OAB condition is escalating as our population ages [2]. Pharmacotherapy is most appropriately first-line treatment for OAB, but the several drugs currently available do not cure the condition for most patients. Many patients discontinue drug therapy because of intolerable side effects, expense, or lack of long-term adherence. Alternative treatments are needed for patients who are unable to tolerate pharmacotherapy or who do not derive the desired benefits.

Historical context

It is hard to believe that little more than 5 to 10 years ago, clinicians had few treatment options to offer refractory OAB patients. Generic oxybutynin and the tricyclic antidepressant class of drugs were the typical agents of choice. Tolterodine arrived on the market only in 2000. When the available pharmacotherapy failed to offer benefit, some clinicians offered augmentation enterocystoplasty as a last resort. Given the scope of potential short-term and long-term complications after such major intestinal reconstructive surgery, most patients opted for diapers and catheters instead [3].

Meanwhile, animal model research during the latter half of the twentieth century helped to explain the neurophysiologic wiring of lower urinary tract control [4,5]. Some early clinical experimentation with functional electrical stimulation proved promising for control of urinary urge incontinence. As nonsurgical modalities, such techniques have used surface electrodes, anal and vaginal plug electrodes [6–8], and dorsal penile nerve electrodes [9,10]. Overall, however, such noninvasive modalities of stimulation have been limited by the intensive nature of the multiple treatment sessions and have proved less reliable at achieving and maintaining response.

The anatomic dissections and work of Tanagho and Schmidt [11] in the 1980s led to the development of a more invasive in situ modality of direct electrical stimulation of the sacral nerve root. This technique was the progenitor of the present-day sacral neuromodulation technique in widespread use. This technology is synonymously referred to in the literature as "sacral nerve stimulation" (SNS).

SNS capitalizes on the same principles as functional electrical stimulation; however, the close contact with the nerve root and the continuous electrical stimulation appear to offer the distinct advantage of more durable, consistent control of lower urinary tract dysfunction. This minimally invasive technology, which requires subcutaneous implantation of the electrode and pulse generator, is described later in the article.

How does sacral nerve stimulation work?

Pilot clinical trial data of the early 1990s led to US Food and Drug Administration (FDA) approval of the sacral neuromodulation device implantation in 1997. SNS has proved to be an

This project is supported by NIH grant 1K23 DK 62726-01/NIDDK.
    * Corresponding author.
    E-mail address: lengww@upmc.edu (W.W. Leng).

doi:10.1016/j.ucl.2006.06.009

effective, minimally invasive urologic surgical technique for the treatment of diverse lower urinary tract disorders; namely, refractory urinary urge incontinence and idiopathic voiding dysfunction or retention. Naturally, one must question how a single electrode stimulation of the third sacral foramen nerve root can serve such disparate clinical indications. Indeed, how can the same technique be used to control urge incontinence in one patient and to restore micturition in another patient who has idiopathic urinary retention?

Although this article is focused on the ability of SNS to treat OAB symptoms, it is helpful to revisit the pertinent neuroanatomy and neurophysiology of lower urinary tract functions. Understanding the fundamental blueprint of the central nervous system controls of micturition is essential to appreciating how SNS can treat a seemingly wide range of lower urinary tract dysfunctions. More details regarding the theorized range of mechanisms of action of SNS can be found elsewhere [12].

The micturition blueprint

Normal micturition is dependent on multiple overlapping neural pathways in the central nervous system. These pathways coalesce to perform three major functions: amplification, coordination, and timing [13]. The nervous system control of the lower urinary tract must be able to amplify weak smooth muscle activity to provide sustained increases of bladder contractility sufficient to empty the bladder. Likewise, the bladder and urethral sphincter function must be coordinated to allow the sphincter to open during micturition but to remain closed at all other times. Timing reflects the volitional nature of control over voiding that occurs with toilet training in human development. This control affords us the ability to initiate voiding over a wide range of bladder volumes.

In this regard, the bladder is a unique visceral organ that exhibits predominately voluntary rather than involuntary (autonomic) neural regulation. A number of important reflex mechanisms contribute to the storage and elimination of urine and modulate the voluntary control of micturition [14]. As an autonomically regulated organ, the bladder is also unusual in the sense that it remains in a "turned off" mode for most of the time. Thus, it behaves in a distinctively different manner than other visceral organs such as the heart, blood vessels, and gastrointestinal tract—all of which receive tonic autonomic regulation. When volitional desire

to urinate occurs, the bladder "turns on" in an "all-or-none" manner to eliminate urine.

The ability to "turn on" micturition in a switch-like fashion is facilitated by positive feedback loops in the micturition reflex pathway. During the micturitional amplification stage, bladder afferent activity stimulates sufficient efferent excitatory input to the bladder, which in turn initiates a bladder contraction. This positive feedback system, mediated in part by supraspinal parasympathetic pathways to the pontine micturition center, is a very effective mechanism for promoting efficient bladder emptying and for minimizing residual urine.

This positive feedback mechanism, however, can also pose as a potentially significant liability. In the presence of neuropathology, the positive feedback system may escape central inhibitory controls or may excessively sensitize bladder afferent signaling. The overall result of such a loss of "checks and balance" is the emergence of bladder hyperactivity and random urge incontinence.

Afferent and efferent pathways

Efferent outflow to the lower urinary tract can be activated by spinal afferent pathways and by input from the brain. Afferent signaling input from the lower urinary tract is key to modulating voiding function. Such afferent signaling arises from two main sources: (1) the pelvic visceral organs and (2) somatic afferent pathways by way of the pudendal nerves from the perineal muscle and skin. Although micturition control is commonly perceived as a primarily autonomic-driven circuit, somatic afferent pathways transmit important feedback from the genital organs, urethra, prostate, vagina, anal canal, and skin, which can modulate voiding function [13–15].

Bladder afferent nerves are critical for sending signals of bladder fullness and discomfort to the brain to initiate the micturition reflex. The bladder afferent pathways are composed of two types of axons: small myelinated A-delta fibers and unmyelinated C-fibers. A-delta fibers transmit signals mainly from mechanoreceptors that detect bladder fullness or wall tension. The C-fibers, on the other hand, mainly detect noxious signals and initiate painful sensations. The bladder C-fiber nociceptors perform a similar function and signal the central nervous system whenever an infection or irritative condition exists in the bladder. C-fiber bladder afferents also have reflex functions to facilitate or trigger voiding [16,17], which can be viewed as a bodily defense mechanism to eliminate irritants or bacteria from the lower urinary tract. The C-fiber bladder afferents have been implicated in the triggering of reflex bladder hyperactivity associated with neurologic disorders such as spinal cord injury and multiple sclerosis.

Bladder hyperactivity and urinary incontinence presumably occur as the consequence of loss of voluntary control of voiding and the re-emergence of primitive voiding reflex circuitry. Such primitive voiding reflexes are hypothesized to have been normal neonatal reflex patterns that in time became suppressed with postnatal development. Alternatively, new reflex circuits could arise as a consequence of abnormal C-fiber afferent sensitization [18].

Under normal conditions, the latter are thought to be mechanoinsensitive and unresponsive to bladder distension (hence the name "silent" C-fibers). As a consequence of neurologic or inflammatory diseases or possibly during the aging process, however, the silent C-fibers may become sensitized to bladder distension and thus trigger unwanted micturition reflexes [17]. This type of bladder hyperactivity could theoretically be suppressed by blocking C-fiber afferent activity or by interrupting reflex pathways in the spinal cord by SNS.

Latent inhibitory pathways

To serve as a balance to the micturition blueprint design, nature has provided other latent mechanisms for inhibitory modulation of the micturition reflex. These more primitive mechanisms reside in the spinal cord and can be awakened by stimulation of various somatic and visceral afferent nerves [5,19]. The spinal organization of these inhibitory mechanisms has been elucidated by electrophysiologic studies in animals [20,21]. The authors hypothesize that these modulatory mechanisms can be reactivated by SNS in the treatment of the OAB condition (Fig. 1).

Experimental data from animals [22] have shown that sacral preganglionic outflow to the urinary bladder receives inhibitory inputs from various somatic and visceral afferents and from a recurrent inhibitory pathway [4,5,19]. The experiments have also provided information about the organization of these inhibitory mechanisms [20,21]. Electrical stimulation of somatic afferents in the pudendal nerve elicits inhibitory mechanisms [18]. This result is supported by the finding that interneurons in the sacral autonomic nucleus

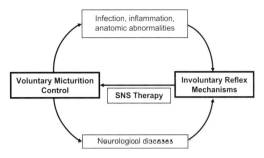

Fig. 1. Conceptual diagram shows that SNS modulates the balance of volitional and reflex pathways controlling micturition.

exhibit firing correlated with bladder activity and demonstrate inhibition by activation of somatic afferent pathways. This electrical stimulation of somatic afferent nerves in the sacral spinal roots could inhibit reflex bladder hyperactivity mediated by spinal or supraspinal pathways.

Pelvic floor electrical stimulation

In addition to the strong evidence from animal research that identified somatic afferent modulation of bladder and urethral reflexes, there are also data from clinical physiologic studies. As previously mentioned, functional electrical stimulation offers a favorable nonsurgical treatment for many patients who have detrusor instability. Stimulation techniques typically use surface electrodes, anal and vaginal plug electrodes, and dorsal penile nerve electrodes.

Such clinical research reinforces the view that stimulation of sacral afferent circuits can modify bladder and urethral sphincter reflexes. The success of pelvic floor electrical stimulation therapy relies on convergence of common visceral and somatic sensory innervation pathways in the central nervous system [23]. By stimulating somatic afferent pathways, it is possible to block the processing of visceral afferent signals being delivered to the same region of the spinal cord. Another example of this principle is the technique of posterior tibial nerve stimulation. With percutaneous electrical stimulation of this nerve or its dermatome, it is possible to block sensory afferent inputs from the bladder [24]. Ohlsson and associates [8] reported encouraging success using electrical somatic nerve stimulation with transvaginal probes in women and transrectal probes in men. Despite a documented average 45% increase in bladder capacity, only one half of their patients reported a 30% decrease in the frequency of micturition. Fall [6] also reported favorable long-term results of vaginal electrical stimulation in the treatment of refractory detrusor instability and stress urinary incontinence. Seventy three percent of the women who had detrusor instability became asymptomatic during treatment, whereas 45% remained free of symptoms after discontinuation of therapy. Many patients, however, required up to 6 months of therapy before benefit was apparent.

Sacral nerve stimulation suppression of bladder hyperactivity

Several reflex mechanisms may be involved in the SNS suppression of bladder hyperactivity. Afferent pathways projecting to the sacral cord can inhibit bladder reflexes in animals and humans by way of two pathways: (1) inhibition of the sacral interneuronal transmission and (2) direct inhibition of bladder preganglionic neurons of the efferent limb of the micturition reflex circuit (Fig. 2). The source of afferent input may be somatic, visceral, or both; namely, sphincter muscles, distal colon, rectum, anal canal, vagina, uterine cervix, and cutaneous innervation from the perineum. Of the two aforementioned mechanisms responsible for somatic and visceral afferent inhibition of bladder reflexes, the most common mechanism at play in SNS is believed to be the suppression of interneuronal transmission in the bladder reflex pathway [16,25].

It is assumed that this inhibition occurs, in part, on the ascending limb of the micturition reflex and therefore blocks the transfer of signaling input from the bladder to the pontine micturition center. This action prevents involuntary (reflex) micturition but does not necessarily suppress voluntary voiding. This is the clinical scenario typically observed in SNS therapy of OAB. The preservation of volitional voiding function suggests that the descending excitatory efferent pathways from the brain to the sacral parasympathetic preganglionic neurons are not inhibited.

Targeting the descending excitatory efferent pathways is much more effective in turning off micturition reflexes because it directly suppresses firing within the spinal cord motor outflow. This suppression can be induced by electrical stimulation of the pudendal nerve or by mechanical stimulation of the anal canal and distal bowel. As alluded to, however, such stimulation is also expected to nonselectively block voluntary and involuntary voiding. Therefore, this inhibitory pathway appears to play a lesser role in the explanation of SNS mechanism of action. As a large body of experience has shown, SNS performed for voiding dysfunction or OAB syndrome typically allows patients to retain normal voiding mechanisms.

The authors hypothesize that SNS effects depend on electrical stimulation of somatic afferent axons in the spinal roots, which in turn modulate voiding and continence reflex pathways in the central nervous system. The afferent system is the most likely target because beneficial effects can be elicited at intensities of stimulation that do not activate movements of striated muscles [26–28].

Indications for sacral nerve stimulation

Currently, the InterStim (Medtronic, Minneapolis, MN) device has approval from the FDA for the following indications: (1) refractory urge incontinence, (2) refractory urgency and frequency, and (3) idiopathic urinary retention. As a minimally invasive, outpatient urologic procedure, SNS has demonstrated long-term efficacy and safety. Later in this article, the reported outcomes and complications data are summarized.

In addition to the previously mentioned FDA-approved indications, there is a growing body of clinical experience that suggests the value of SNS technology for other ancillary applications. For example, small case series have shown that SNS can improve lower urinary tract symptoms associated with multiple sclerosis and incomplete

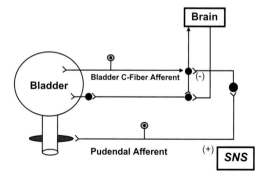

Fig. 2. Stimulation of multiple afferent nerve pathways can inhibit the micturition reflex.

spinal cord lesions [29,30] in addition to interstitial cystitis and pelvic floor pain [31].

Patient selection

It is common practice to begin empiric conservative treatment of clinical OAB symptoms. Typically, conservative therapy for this condition encompasses dedicated trials of combination anticholinergic pharmacotherapy, pelvic floor physiotherapy, and behavioral modification. When it becomes apparent that conservative therapy has failed, the patient should undergo urodynamic testing to objectively characterize the lower urinary tract symptoms.

A thorough bladder diary completed by the patient adds another dimension of documentation regarding the severity of urgency/frequency symptoms and the number of leak episodes. The diary also offers insight into the amount and timing of fluid intake. Because the patient's subjective symptom reporting is central to the success or failure of SNS testing, a well documented bladder diary is critical to patient selection.

Not every appropriate candidate for SNS will derive benefit. It is unfortunate that no current, reliable predictors are available to determine which subset of candidates may achieve response. The InterStim procedure, therefore, must be conducted with a preliminary test phase.

Contraindications

The usual contraindications encompass any patient who fails to achieve an appropriate symptom response to test stimulation. Likewise, clinical judgment must dictate whether a patient is capable of operating the neurostimulator device. Other potential urologic contraindications include conditions of bladder outlet obstruction such as benign prostatic hypertrophy, urethral stricture, or cancer.

Another important contraindication, not often mentioned in the urologic literature, pertains to any subsequent use of diathermy. This therapeutic modality involves the generation of local heat in targeted body tissues by high-frequency electromagnetic radiation, electric currents, or ultrasonic waves. Traditionally, diathermy has been used by a range of health care providers including physical therapists, chiropractors, dentists, and sports therapists in efforts to promote wound healing and to relieve muscle pain and spasms.

This modality is now being used more and more in minimally invasive surgery. Any mode of diathermy can theoretically transfer energy through the implant device and cause severe local tissue injury due to heating at the tissue/device interface. Such tissue injury could lead to permanent injury or even death. Regardless of whether the implanted neurostimulation device is turned off, its presence still poses a risk of injury to surrounding tissue and of device failure. Further details can be found at the manufacturer's Web site: http://www.medtronic.com/neuro/interstim/ interstim_warning.html.

Techniques

Percutaneous nerve evaluation

Traditionally, a test trial period known as percutaneous nerve evaluation (PNE) was performed in the office setting using local anesthesia. After the temporary test electrode was placed in the third sacral foramen, the lead was then secured to the skin and connected to an external pulse generator. Three to 5 days of test stimulation followed, with the completion of another bladder diary. Based on this short-term follow-up evaluation, the patients who achieved sufficient symptom improvement had the temporary lead removed and proceeded to a scheduled operative permanent neuromodulator device implantation. With refinement of the operative techniques over time, what once involved an open surgical incision and exposure of the paramedian sacrum has evolved into a minimally invasive, percutaneous procedure [32].

The PNE test stimulation, however, offers a sizeable degree of false-positive and false-negative responses in up to 40% of patients [33]. Because of inconsistent test responses and theoretic temporary lead migration, the development of a tined lead permanent electrode offers another option.

Tined lead electrode

The advent of the tined lead modification (Fig. 3) in 2002 brought a number of technical improvements: (1) a sutureless anchoring system that allowed for a minimal surgical incision; (2) minimal incisions allowed for the procedure to be performed under a combination of intravenous sedation and supplemental local anesthesia, and (3) short-acting sedation allowed for intraoperative testing of patient sensory response to

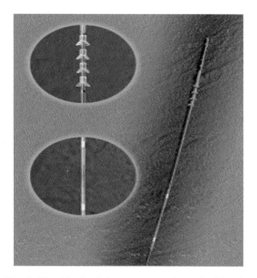

Fig. 3. Tined leads of the permanent electrode. (Reprinted with the permission of Medtronic, Inc. © 2006.)

stimulation. These advantages have led to the increasing popularity of the staged permanent electrode placement. Instead of the usual PNE described earlier, many clinicians are opting to perform the stage 1 test stimulation in the outpatient operating room setting using the tined lead permanent electrode. Proper positioning with the percutaneous approach can be readily confirmed with fluoroscopic guidance (Fig. 4).

Aside from the logistic advantages, the tined lead staged procedures also offer the ability to prolong the testing interval from a few days to a few weeks. With less chance of electrode migration and a longer test interval, one can anticipate a higher likelihood of a positive response to SNS. A recent prospective randomized trial compared the outcomes of one- versus two-stage techniques [34]. Although this study was relatively small, the findings suggested that the two-stage method had a higher short-term and long-term success rate. Although the two-stage implant added an additional direct cost of 1941 Euro per patient, the investigators contended that the lower revision and failure rates rendered the two methods cost-equivalent.

If a satisfactory motor and sensory response to stimulation is achieved (Table 1) with stage 1 testing, then it is appealing to use the same successful electrode as part of the definitive implantation device. If the patient does not achieve any benefit from SNS, then the tined lead electrode and its temporary percutaneous wires can be easily disconnected and removed at a second brief operating room visit.

The final implantable InterStim system is comprised of a battery-powered neurostimulator, an extension cable, and the tined lead with quadripolar electrodes (Fig. 5). At the second stage of permanent implantation, the pulse generator is placed within a subcutaneous pocket of the superior buttock. Subsequent adjustments of the stimulator impulse settings can be accomplished easily and noninvasively with the use of a remote electronic programming device [11,35–37].

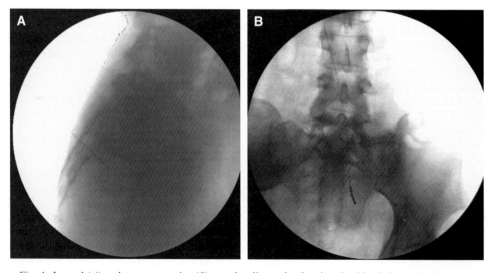

Fig. 4. Lateral (*A*) and anteroposterior (*B*) sacral radiographs showing tined lead electrode placement.

Table 1
Reflex responses to sacral nerve root stimulation

Nerve Root	Pelvic Floor	Ipsilateral Lower Extremity	Sensation
S2	Anal sphincter contraction	Lateral leg rotation, contraction of toes and foot	Vaginal or proximal penile contraction
S3	"Bellows" response of pelvic floor, bladder and urethral sphincter contraction	Great toe plantar flexion	"Pulling" in rectum, variable sensations in labia, tip of penis or scrotum
S4	"Bellows" response of pelvic floor	None	"Pulling" in rectum

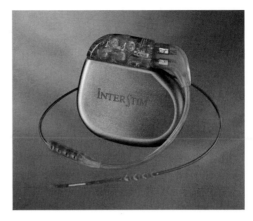

Fig. 5. SNS InterStim permanent implantable device components. (Reprinted with the permission of Medtronic, Inc. © 2006.)

Reported outcomes and complications

Large case series and randomized controlled trials of the SNS device have been ongoing since the early 1990s. The collective efficacy data demonstrate that approximately 70% of patients who undergo SNS testing for urgency, frequency, or urge incontinence achieve success compared with the 4% within comparable control groups (Tables 2–4) [38–41]. It is important to clearly define "success" for the patient as "greater than 50% improvement of symptoms." Certainly, there will be occasions where a patient cannot readily judge the degree of symptom relief attained with the SNS device. In such a situation, a 24-hour trial with the stimulator device turned off makes the determination clearer for the patient and the physician. Multiple studies have shown that deactivation of the stimulator device results in rapid return to baseline symptoms for most patients. Similarly, reactivation of the same device leads to prompt return of symptom control [39,41,42].

In an overall review of adverse events reported from 27 studies in the literature, Brazzelli and colleagues [38] noted an overall surgical revision rate of 33%. Most commonly, reoperation was

Table 2
Sacral nerve stimulation therapy outcomes for urgency frequency

Author	Type of study	N=	Technique	F/U (mo)	Reported outcome variables	Overall conclusion
Everaert 2002 abstract	RCT	22	PNE vs staged implant	12	• +129 ml bladder capacity • −3 daily voids	
Hassouna 2000	RCT	25	PNE	6–24	• +91 ml bladder capacity • −7.6 mean daily voids • +101 ml mean void volume • −0.4 urgency rank	• 56% improved at least 50 percent at 6 months
Siegel 2000	Prospective cohort	29	PNE	24	• −7.1 mean daily voids • +92.5 ml mean void volume	• 56% improved at least 50 percent • Urge severity improved 69%

Table 3
Sacral nerve stimulation therapy outcomes for urge incontinence

Author	Type of study	N=	Technique	F/U (mo)	Reported outcome variables	Overall conclusion
Everaert 2004	Randomized trial	8	One-stage	12–24	• +101 ml void volume • 0 leaks/day at 24 mo • −3 mean daily voids	Failures positively related to one-stage implant, and negatively related to age
		9	Two-staged	24	• + 126 ml void volume • 0 leaks/day at 24 mo • −3 mean daily voids	
Weil 2000	RCT	38	PNE	6–36	• −88% mean leak episodes • −90% mean pad use • + 39% bladder capacity	• 56% dry in implant group • 4% dry in controls • 33% improved at least 50 percent
Schmidt 1999	RCT	58	PNE	6–36	• −7.1 mean daily leak episodes • −5.1 mean daily pad use • + 143 ml bladder capacity	• 47% dry • 29% improved at least 50 percent
Siegel 2000	Prospective cohort	41	PNE	36	• −5.6 mean daily leak episodes • −2.3 mean heavy leak episodes • −3.3 mean daily pad use	• 46% dry • 13% improved at least 50 percent
Spinelli 2001	Registry Retrospective	84 42	PNE	 41	 • 42% had <8 voids daily • 42% had 8–12 voids daily • 18% had > 12 voids daily	 • 39% dry • 23% less than one daily leak episode
	Prospective	42		6–18	• −4.3 mean daily leak episodes • 84% had < 8 voids daily at 6 months	• 65% dry at 6 mo • 43% dry at 18 mo
Bosch 2002	Prospective cohort	44	PNE	47	• −4.2 mean daily pad use • −5.8 mean daily leak episodes • −4.9 mean daily voids • +47 ml void volume • +76 mean bladder capacity	• 40% dry • 20% improved at least 50 percent

performed for the following device-related reasons: (1) to relocate the pulse generator because of pain, (2) to revise lead placement because of inadvertent lead migration, or (3) to remove the entire device due to local infection.

The introduction of the tined lead implantation system has simplified the overall operative procedure. What was once a paramedian incision and dissection down to fascial anchoring of the electrode has evolved into a percutaneous lead insertion guided by fluoroscopy. In addition, the tines theoretically help to secure the desired lead positioning within the soft tissues. The reported incidence of lead migration with the earlier technique was significant (range, 11.8%–16%) and would often lead to loss of stimulation efficacy [43]. In addition, relocating the implantable pulse generator from its original position within the lower abdomen to an upper buttock site has decreased the incidence of pain and infection at the device location from 42% to 16% [44]. Reported adverse events, however, appear to be

Table 4
Sacral nerve stimulation implant: reported complications rate

Authors	Type of study	N=	F/U (mo)	Incid (%)	Reported complication	Notes
Hassouna 2000	Prospective cohort	219	12			Based upon pooled data
				15.3	• Pain at implant site	
				9	• New pain	
				8.4	• Lead migration	
				6.1	• Infection	
				5.5	• Transient electrical shock	
				5.4	• Pain at lead site	
				3	• Adverse change in bowel function	
				1.7	• Technical problems	
				1.6	• Device malfunction	
				1	• Change in menses	
				0.6	• Adverse change in voiding	
				0.5	• Persistent skin irritation	
				0.5	• Suspected nerve injury	
				0.5	• Device rejection	
				9.5	• Other	
				33.3	• Surgical revision	
Schmidt 1999	RCT	157	6–36			Based upon pooled data
				15.9	• Pain at implant site	
				19.1	• Pain at lead site	
				7	• Lead migration	
				5.7	• infection	
				32.5	• Surgical revision	• Surgical revision did not prevent favorable outcome

readily corrected by device revision or, as a last resort, device explantation. To date, no major neurologic complications have been reported [41].

Quality-of-life impact

The quality-of-life research in the area of the OAB condition continues to burgeon. Questionnaires, generic (Short-Form 36 Health Survey) and condition specific (Incontinence Impact Questionnaire), are being used more and more in the evaluation of OAB therapies. The scrutiny of potential benefits of sacral neuromodulation for overall patient well-being is no exception. Some investigators have recently reported significant global improvement of patient perception of quality of life with respect to SNS outcomes [45–47].

Summary

Overall, efficacy data from a collective body of global clinical experience supports the conclusion

that an estimated 70% of patients who receive SNS therapy become dry or show substantial (>50%) improvement of their otherwise refractory OAB symptoms. The cited randomized controlled trials [38–42] further support this efficacy, given that the control groups (usual conservative therapy) experienced only a 4% benefit [42]. The safety profile of the implantation procedure remains consistent over the increasing length of follow-up since the device's introduction to the clinical market. The relatively high revision rate of 33% has been a relative concern; however, since the late 1990s, the revision rate appears to have dropped significantly [48]. One can speculate that device modifications and growing clinician experience with the technology and procedure have played important roles.

SNS therapy has evolved into one of the most widely accepted treatment modalities in the arena of neurourology. The authors believe that SNS activates or "resets" the somatic afferent inputs that play a pivotal role in the modulation of sensory processing for micturition reflex pathways in the spinal cord. Lower urinary tract symptoms of the OAB syndrome can be suppressed by one or more pathways (ie, by direct inhibition of bladder preganglionic neurons or by inhibition of interneuronal transmission in the afferent limb of the micturition reflex). When conservative treatments for OAB symptoms fail, this minimally invasive technology offers a safe, reliable, and durable treatment for lower urinary tract dysfunction.

References

[1] Coyne KS, Payne C, Bhattacharyya SK, et al. The impact of urinary urgency and frequency on health-related quality of life in overactive bladder: results from a national community survey. Value Health 2004;7(4):455–63.

[2] Stewart WF, Van Rooyen JB, Cundiff GW, et al. Prevalence and burden of overactive bladder in the United States. World J Urol 2003;20(6):327–36.

[3] Schmidt RA. Treatment of unstable bladder. Urology 1991;37:28–32.

[4] de Groat WC, Ryall RW. The identification and antidromic responses of sacral preganglionic parasympathetic neurons. J Physiol 1968;196:533–77.

[5] de Groat WC, Ryall RW. Recurrent inhibition in sacral parasympathetic pathways to the bladder. J Physiol 1968;196:579–91.

[6] Fall M. Electrical pelvic floor stimulation for the control of detrusor instability. Neurourol Urodyn 1985;4:329–35.

[7] Janez J, Plevnik S, Suhet P. Urethral and bladder responses to anal electrical stimulation. J Urol 1979; 122:192–4.

[8] Ohlsson BL, Fall M, Frankenbers-Sommar S. Effects of external and direct pudendal nerve maximal electrical stimulation in the treatment of the uninhibited overactive bladder. Br J Urol 1989;64:374–80.

[9] Walter JS, Wheeler JS, Robinson CJ, et al. Inhibiting the hyperreflexic bladder with electrical stimulation in a spinal animal model. Neurourol Urodyn 1993;12:241–52.

[10] Wheeler JS, Walter JS. Bladder inhibition by dorsal penile nerve stimulation in spinal cord injured patients. J Urol 1992;147:100–3.

[11] Tanagho EA, Schmidt RA. Electrical stimulation in the clinical management of the neurogenic bladder. J Urol 1988;140:1331–9.

[12] Leng WW, Chancellor MB. How sacral nerve stimulation neuromodulation works. Urol Clin North Am 2005;32(1):11–8.

[13] de Groat WC. Central nervous system control of micturition. In: O'Donnell PD, editor. Urinary incontinence. St. Louis (MO): Mosby; 1997. p. 33–47.

[14] de Groat WC, Araki I, Vizzard MA, et al. Developmental and injury induced plasticity in the micturition reflex pathway. Behav Brain Res 1998; 92:127–40.

[15] Yoshimura N, de Groat WC. Neural control of the lower urinary tract. Int J Urol 1997;4:111–25.

[16] Kruse MN, Noto H, Roppolo JR, et al. Pontine control of the urinary bladder and external urethral sphincter in the rat. Brain Res 1990;532:182–90.

[17] Cheng CI, Ma CP, de Groat WC. Effect of capsaicin on micturition and associated reflexes in rats. Am J Physiol 1993;34:R132–8.

[18] de Groat WC. Changes in the organization of the micturition reflex pathway of the cat after transection of the spinal cord. Exper Neurol 1981;71: 22–5.

[19] de Groat WC. Nervous control of the urinary bladder of the cat. Brain Res 1975;87:201–11.

[20] de Groat WC. Inhibition and excitation of sacral parasympathetic neurons by visceral and cutaneous stimuli in the cat. Brain Res 1971;33:499–503.

[21] de Groat WC. Mechanisms underlying recurrent inhibition in the sacral parasympathetic outflow to the urinary bladder. J Physiol 1976;257:503–13.

[22] de Groat WC. Inhibitory mechanisms in the sacral reflex pathways to the urinary bladder. In: Ryall RW, Kelly JS, editors. Iontophoresis and transmitter mechanisms in the mammalian central nervous system. Amsterdam: Elsevier; 1978. p. 366–8.

[23] Morrison JFB. Neural connections between the lower urinary tract and the spinal cord. In: Torrens M, Morrison JFB, editors. The physiology of the lower urinary tract. London: Springer Verlag; 1987. p. 53–85.

[24] McGuire EJ, Shi-Chun Z, Horwinski R, et al. Treatment of motor and sensory detrusor instability by electrical stimulation. J Urol 1983;129:78–9.

[25] de Groat WC, Theobald RJ. Reflex activation of sympathetic pathways to vesical smooth muscle and parasympathetic ganglia by electrical stimulation of vesical afferents. J Physiol 1976;259:223–7.

[26] Thon WF, Baskin LS, Jonas U, et al. Surgical principles of sacral foramen electrode implantation. World J Urol 1991;9:133–7.

[27] Vodusek DB, Light JK, Liddy JM. Detrusor inhibition induced by stimulation of pudendal nerve afferents. Neurourol Urodyn 1986;5:381–9.

[28] de Groat WC, Kruse MN, Vizzard MA, et al. Modification of urinary bladder function after neural injury. In: Seil F, editor. Advances in neurology: neuronal regeneration, reorganization, and repair, vol. 72. New York: Lippincott-Raven; 1997. p. 347–64.

[29] Bosch JLHR, Groen J. Treatment of refractory urge urinary incontinence with sacral spinal nerve stimulation in multiple sclerosis patients. Lancet 1996;348: 717–9.

[30] Bosch JLHR, Groen J. Neuromodulation: urodynamic effects of sacral (S3) spinal nerve stimulation in patients with detrusor instability or detrusor hyperreflexia. Behav Brain Res 1998;92:141–50.

[31] Bernstein AJ, Peters KM. Expanding indications for neuromodulation. Urol Clin North Am 2005;32(1): 59–63.

[32] Spinelli M, Giardiello G, Gerber M, et al. New sacral neuromodulation lead for percutaneous implantation using local anesthesia: description and first experience. J Urol 2003;170(5):1905–7.

[33] Bosch R, Groen J. Sacral nerve neuromodulation in the treatment of patients with refractory motor urge incontinence: long-term results of a prospective longitudinal study. J Urol 2000;163:1219–22.

[34] Everaert K, Kerckhaert W, Caluwaerts H, et al. A prospective randomized trial comparing the 1-stage with the 2-stage implantation of a pulse generator in patients with pelvic floor dysfunction selected for sacral nerve stimulation. Eur Urol 2004;45:649–54.

[35] Juenemann KP, Lue TF, Schmidt RA, et al. Clinical significance of sacral and pudendal nerve anatomy. J Urol 1988;139:74–80.

[36] Schmidt RA, Tanagho EA. Feasibility of controlled micturition through electric stimulation. Urol Int 1979;34:199–230.

[37] Schmidt RA, Sennm E, Tanagho EA. Functional evaluation of sacral nerve root integrity. Report of a technique. Urology 1990;35:388–92.

[38] Brazzelli M, Murray A, Fraser C, et al. Systematic review of the efficacy and safety of sacral nerve stimulation for urinary urge incontinence and urgency-frequency. J Urol 2006;175(3):835–41.

[39] Schmidt RA, Jonas U, Oleson KA. Sacral nerve stimulation for the treatment of refractory urge incontinence. J Urol 1999;162:352–7.

[40] Spinelli M, Bertapelle P, Cappellano F, et al. Chronic sacral neuromodulation in patients with lower urinary tract symptoms: results from a national register. J Urol 2001;166:541–5.

[41] Hassouna MM, Siegel SW, Nyeholt AA, et al. Sacral neuromodulation in the treatment of urgency-frequency symptoms: a multicentre study on efficacy and safety. J Urol 2000;163:1849–54.

[42] Weil DH, Ruiz-Cerda JL, Eerdmans PH, et al. Sacral root neuromodulation in the treatment of refractory urinary urge incontinence: a prospective randomized clinical trial. Eur Urol 2000;37(2): 161–71.

[43] Siegel SW, Catanzaro F, Dijkema H, et al. Long-term results of a multicenter study on sacral nerve stimulation for treatment of urinary urge incontinence, urgency-frequency, and retention. Urology 2000;56(Suppl 6A):87–91.

[44] Das AK, Siegel S, Rivas DA, et al. Upper buttock placement of sacral neurostimulator results in decreased adverse events and reoperation rates. Proceedings of the 32nd Annual Meeting of the International Continence Society. Heidelberg, Germany, 2002.

[45] Amundsen CL, Webster GD. Sacral neuromodulation in an older, urge-incontinent population. Am J Obstet Gynecol 2002;187(6):1462–5.

[46] Cappellano F, Bertapelle P, Spinelli M, et al. Quality of life assessment in patients who undergo sacral neuromodulation implantation for urge incontinence: an additional tool for evaluating outcome. J Urol 2001;166(6):2277–80.

[47] Shaker HS, Hassouna M. Sacral nerve root neuromodulation: an effective treatment for refractory urge incontinence. J Urol 1998;159:1516–9.

[48] Van Voskuilen AC, Oerlemans DJAJ, Weil EHJ, et al. Long-term results of neuromodulation by sacral nerve stimulation for lower urinary tract symptoms: a retrospective single center study. Eur Urol 2006;49(2):366–72.

ELSEVIER
SAUNDERS

Urol Clin N Am 33 (2006) 503–510

UROLOGIC
CLINICS
of North America

The Case for Bladder Botulinum Toxin Application

Dae Kyung Kim, MD, PhD[a], Catherine A. Thomas, PhD[b],
Christopher Smith, MD[b], Michael B. Chancellor, MD[b],*

[a]Department of Urology, Eulji University School of Medicine, 1306 Dunsandong Seogu, Daejeon, Korea
[b]Department of Urology, University of Pittsburgh School of Medicine, Suite 700, 3471 Fifth Avenue,
Pittsburgh, PA 15213, USA

First isolated by van Ermengem in 1897, botulinum toxin (BoNT) is the most potent biologic toxin known to man [1]. The toxin acts by inhibiting acetylcholine release at the presynaptic cholinergic junction. Clinically, the urologic community initially used commercial preparations of BoNT type A (BoNT-A) to treat spinal cord–injury (SCI) patients suffering from detrusor-sphincter dyssynergia [2–4]. More recently, urologists have injected BoNT-A into the detrusor muscles of patients suffering from overactive bladders of neurogenic or idiopathic etiologies.

There are three commercially available preparations of BoNT; two are of type A neurotoxin and one is of type B. It is important to note that although these BoNTs are produced from the same bacteria, *Clostridium botulinum*, they differ in potency and dose and are therefore not interchangeable.

Standard treatment for neurogenic bladder overactivity involves the use of antimuscarinic medications. Unwanted side effects and lack of efficacy have led to poor long-term compliance with current oral therapies. Newer agents that target sensory fibers (eg, capsaicin and resiniferatoxin [RTX]) have shown early clinical promise but are currently unavailable within the United States market [5]. Short of more invasive surgical procedures (eg, sacral nerve stimulation, sacral rhizotomy, bladder myomectomy, and bladder augmentation), few other options to help treat patients who have neurogenic incontinence have been available.

Neurogenic detrusor overactivity

Adult population

In 1999, Stohrer and colleagues [6] first described the use of BoNT-A to treat neurogenic detrusor overactivity (NDO). Since then, several peer-reviewed articles and abstracts are now available within the scientific community. Schurch and colleagues [7] demonstrated a significant increase in mean maximum bladder capacity (from 296 to 480 mL, $P < .016$) and a significant decrease in mean maximum detrusor voiding pressure (from 65 to 35 cm H_2O, $P < .016$) in 21 patients who had detrusor hyper-reflexia and were injected with BoNT-A. Seventeen of 19 patients were completely continent at 6-week follow-up and were very satisfied with the procedure. In 11 patients followed for 9 months, improvement in urodynamic parameters and incontinence persisted compared with baseline measurements. Del Popolo [8] also demonstrated significant increases in mean bladder capacity (from 240.5 mL to 400 mL) that lasted between 4 and 16 months in 61 patients who had detrusor hyper-reflexia treated with intravesical BoNT-A. Similar clinical responses (range, 4–36 months) from BoNT-A treatment in other autonomic disorders (eg, axillary/palmar hyperhydrosis, gustatory sweating, and sialorrhea) have been described, suggesting that differences in toxin effect or re-innervation may account for the more prolonged clinical responses observed in autonomically versus somatically innervated tissues [9–11].

* Corresponding author.
E-mail address: chancellormb@msx.upmc.edu
(M.B. Chancellor).

0094-0143/06/$ - see front matter © 2006 Elsevier Inc. All rights reserved.
doi:10.1016/j.ucl.2006.06.010

A long-term study in 87 patients who had detrusor hyper-reflexia corroborated the efficacy of intravesical BoNT injection presented in earlier studies [12]. Clinical responses lasted 4 to 14 months, and no adverse effects occurred from treatment. In the largest clinical series presented to date, a multicenter retrospective study examined 200 patients who had neurogenic bladder treated with intravesical BoNT-A injections [13]. At 3- and 9-month follow-up, urodynamic testing revealed significant increases in maximum bladder capacity and significant decreases in voiding pressure. Thus, BoNT-A detrusor injections appear to give durable and significant subjective and objective benefits to patients who have NDO.

Does BoNT bladder injection help with detrusor compliance? A recent study from Thailand [14] reported that BoNT-A injection (300 U) improved bladder compliance in 7 of 10 SCI patients at 6 weeks, but levels returned toward baseline by 36 weeks. This study and other recent studies suggest that decreased bladder compliance can be improved with bladder BoNT injection.

A placebo-controlled phase II prospective randomized study in patients who had NDO supported previous evidence of safety and efficacy of BoNT-A at doses of 200 and 300 U in reducing urinary incontinence episodes by an average of 50%, an effect that lasted for the duration of the 24-week study [15]. Urodynamic parameters, also indicative of efficacy, supported the effectiveness of BoNT-A. Increased bladder capacity, as determined by maximal capacity, was consistently and significantly greater in the BoNT-A–treated patients 2 weeks post treatment through 24 weeks post treatment. Statistically significant superiority to placebo was consistently noted, but the study was not designed to compare the two active doses. There were no significant safety observations noted and no treatment-related adverse events reported in any patients.

Pediatric population

Clinicians have also successfully used intravesical BoNT-A to treat neurogenic bladders in pediatric myelomeningocele patients. Within this patient population, BoNT-A treatment could function as an alternative to bladder augmentation in children who fail conservative treatment including clean catheterization and anticholinergics. Schulte-Baukloh and colleagues [16] demonstrated beneficial effects of BoNT-A detrusor injections in 20 children who had neurogenic bladder. Urodynamics

at 2 to 4 weeks following treatment revealed significant increases (35%) in maximal bladder capacity and significant decreases (41%) in maximal detrusor pressure. Although significant increases in maximum bladder capacity were demonstrated up to 6 months after treatment, no significant difference in maximal detrusor pressure was seen at 3- or 6-month follow-up. A more recent pediatric study with longer follow-up in 15 patients (mean age, 5.8 years) supports earlier studies by demonstrating a 118% increase in maximal bladder capacity ($P < .001$) and a 46% decrease in mean maximal detrusor pressure ($P < .001$) following BoNT-A injection [17]. Moreover, the clinical effects of BoNT-A lasted a mean of 10.5 months and were similar after repeated injection.

Botulinum toxin type A versus resiniferatoxin

Investigators prospectively analyzed the effects of intravesical RTX versus BoNT-A in 25 patients who had NDO [18]. Although patients benefited urodynamically and clinically from either treatment, at 18-month follow-up, BoNT-A injections led to significantly greater reductions in the frequency of daily incontinence episodes (from 4.8 to 0.7 following BoNT-A versus 5.4 to 2.0 following RTX treatment) and in the maximum pressure of uninhibited detrusor contractions. In addition, patients treated with BoNT-A experienced significantly greater increases in maximal bladder capacity (from 212 to 451 mL versus 223 to 328 mL) and in the volume threshold to induce an uninhibited detrusor contraction. Moreover, the clinical response to BoNT-A was more durable than it was to RTX (the mean duration of response following BoNT-A injection was 6.8 months compared with 51.6 days following RTX instillation).

Effects of repeated botulinum toxin type A injections

Chemical denervation effect of BoNT-A is overcome with passage of time. It is the combination of temporary sprouting and reactivation (ability to release acetylcholine and possibly other biomessengers) of the original nerve terminal that is responsible for the termination of therapeutic activity (Box 1). In vivo experiments on striated muscle of mice have shown that after BoNT injection, newly formed nerve sprouts allow detectable neuromuscular transmission 8 to 28 days after injection, when the release of acetylcholine at the original nerve ending is still blocked by BoNT [19].

Box 1. Botulinum toxin mechanisms of action

At the motor nerve terminal, BoNT induces a temporary chemodenervation through the following steps:

1. The toxin binds to acceptors on cholinergic terminals.
2. The molecule is internalized into its own vesicle in the cytoplasm of nerve endings.
3. When it is inside the nerve, BoNT interferes with the exocytosis of cholinergic vesicles, which leads to chemodenervation and reduced muscular contractions.
4. BoNT cleaving–specific proteins (SNAP-25 for BoNT-A and VAMP for BoNT type B) are responsible for docking and fusion of the acetylcholine vesicle to the presynaptic membrane, which in turn interferes with neurotransmitter release and causes muscle relaxation.
5. Over time, terminal sprouting occurs. These sprouts touch down and form transient low-level neuromuscular junctions that release acetylcholine.
6. Finally, the original functional endplate is re-established and sprouts regress. At this point, symptoms will return in some patients.

It is the combination of temporary sprouting and reactivation (the ability to release acetylcholine and possibly other biomessengers) of the original nerve terminal that is responsible for the termination of therapeutic activity.

When the effect of toxin is counteracted by collateral axonal sprouts, a repeated injection of toxin is needed to maintain clinical improvements. Can the repeated injection keep the same efficacy of the first injection? There are several possibilities that may cause a diminished response to repeated injections. First, BoNT may trigger an immune response to produce antibodies that could neutralize the effect of BoNT. Of the several factors facilitating immune responses that have been reported, it has mainly been higher doses and shorter intervals between doses that have contributed to the development of clinical tolerance [20]. Therefore, it is recommended that the minimum effective dose should be used and that repeated injections should be given no more frequently than every 10 to 12 weeks. Current formulation containing less protein contents per unit toxin has proved to have less immunogenic potential. Jankovic and colleagues [21] compared the results when patients treated for cervical dystonia were given the original formulation of BoNT-A (25 ng protein/100 U) or the current formulation of BoNT-A (5 ng of protein/100 U). Blocking antibodies were detected in 4 of 42 (9.5%) patients treated only with the original BoNT-A but were not found in any of the 119 patients treated exclusively with the current BoNT-A ($P < .004$). The second possibility relates to a reactive increase in target intracellular protein production in response to successive injections. This phenomenon has been demonstrated in mice even after single injections [22]. Lastly, it has been suggested that there is some possibility of decreasing bladder compliance due to microscarring of injection sites caused by multiple injections. Haferkamp and colleagues [23], however, reported that no statistically significant change was found in the ultrastructure of the detrusor muscle before or after BoNT injection.

Grosse and colleagues [24] evaluated the effectiveness of repeated detrusor injections of BoNT-A. A total of 49 patients who had refractory NDO received between two and five injections of BoNT-A. The investigators found significant and similar reductions in detrusor overactivity and the use of anticholinergic medication, in addition to significant increases in bladder capacity and compliance after the first and the second injection with BoNT-A. The average interval between injections was 11 months. Schulte-Baukloh and colleagues [25] reported their review of 10 children who had NDO and who received at least three BoNT-A injections. The toxin injections were given an average of every 7.8 months (range, 4–18 months). The mean injection interval in a given patient was between 6.3 ± 1.5 months and 9.6 ± 4.2 months. Urodynamic parameters measured 6 months after each injection showed objective improvement with repeated BoNT-A detrusor injections.

Idiopathic detrusor overactivity

The encouraging results of BoNT bladder injections in patients who had NDO sparked an interest within the urologic community for using this agent to treat patients who have idiopathic detrusor overactivity (IDO).

Radziszewski and associates [26] reported favorably on the effects of intravesical BoNT-A injections in a pilot study of patients who had IDO or functional outlet obstruction. Following intravesical or sphincteric BoNT-A injections, patients demonstrated resolution of incontinence and improved voiding efficiency, respectively. Zermann and colleagues [27] presented their experience with intravesical BoNT-A injection in seven patients who had severe urgency-frequency syndrome refractory to anticholinergic therapy or electrical stimulation. In contrast to other studies involving intravesical injections of BoNT-A, the investigators targeted the trigone and bladder base with five to seven injections of 50 U, 100 U, or 200 U of BoNT-A. Four of seven patients responded to treatment, with decreases in frequency and increased bladder capacity. No mention is made of vesicoureteral reflux as a complication of treatment.

Loch and colleagues [28] presented their BoNT-A experience in 30 patients who had neurogenic and non-neurogenic treatment-resistant urge incontinence. Significant improvement was noted in 20 of 30 patients, with decreases in frequency and a 50% to 100% reduction in pad usage, although differences in responses between neurogenic and non-neurogenic patients were not quantified. Finally, Smith and colleagues [29] found comparable decreases in voiding frequency and incontinence episodes following BoNT-A treatment in 80% (8/10) of overactive bladder patients and 73% (8/11) of neurogenic patients. These small studies suggest that bladder injection with BoNT-A can reliably increase functional bladder capacity and decrease urge incontinence in patients who have refractory IDO.

Rapp and colleagues [30] recently presented the largest series of patients who had detrusor overactivity treated with bladder BoNT injection. Thirty-five patients who had refractory overactive bladder symptoms were treated with 300 U of BoNT-A detrusor injections. Patient response to treatment was assessed using the Incontinence Impact Questionnaire (IIQ)-7 and the Urinary Distress Inventory (UDI)-6. At 3-week follow-up, mean IIQ and UDI symptom scores decreased significantly by 28% and 24%, respectively. Symptom improvement persisted in 14 patients followed up to 6 months after treatment. In addition, pad usage decreased from a mean of 3.9 to 1.8 in these 14 patients.

Werner and colleagues [31] reported a prospective nonrandomized study of BoNT injection (100-U) in urge incontinence patients who had IDO resistant to conventional treatment. Of 26 women included in the study, 14 were dry after 4 weeks, 13 of 20 were dry after 12 weeks, and 3 of 5 were dry after 36 weeks. Only 2 failed to respond. There were no other complications other than nine urinary tract infections within the 51 follow-up visits.

Recently, two prospective studies directly compared the responses to intradetrusor injections of BoNT-A in patients who had IDO or NDO. Kessler and colleagues [32] assessed the effects in 22 consecutive patients (11 NDO and 11 IDO) who had resistance to anticholinergics. These patients were injected with 300 U of toxin into the detrusor, and clinical and urodynamic parameters were assessed before and after BoNT injections. In both groups, median daytime frequency, median nocturia, and median number of used pads decreased significantly. There was a significant increase in median maximum cystometric capacity, median bladder compliance, and median postvoid residual. The effect of BoNT-A injections lasted for a median of 5 months in both groups. There was no significant difference in IDO versus NDO with respect to clinical and urodynamic parameters assessed before and after BoNT-A injections.

Popat and colleagues [33] evaluated the comparable efficacy of BoNT in 44 patients who had spinal NDO and in 31 patients who had IDO. These investigators used a different BoNT dose for each group: 300 U for NDO and 200 U for IDO. At 16 weeks after injection, maximum cystometric capacity increased from 229.1 ± 24.8 to 427.0 ± 26.9 mL in the NDO group ($P < .0001$) and from 193.6 ± 24.0 to 327.1 ± 36.1 mL in the IDO group ($P = .0008$). Frequency, urgency, and urge incontinence were decreased in both groups, but in patients who had NDO, percentage improvement in urgency was greater at 4 weeks (78. 2% versus 56.3%, $P = .019$) and at 16 weeks (78.3% versus 50.7%, $P = .013$). The investigators concluded that patients who have intractable IDO respond with equally significant improvements in urodynamic and lower urinary tract symptom parameters as those who have spinal NDO, despite the lower dose of toxin used.

BoNT type B has also been used in the overactive bladder population, and its effects were described in a study of 15 patients treated with detrusor injections [34]. Investigators found that

14 of 15 patients responded to BoNT type B treatment with a mean decrease in daily micturition episodes of 5.27 ($P < .001$). The duration of response lasted between 19 and 98 days and correlated with toxin dose (eg, 2500–15,000 U); however, even the longest response to BoNT type B injection was of much shorter duration than the 6-month subjective and objective responses to BoNT-A injection demonstrated in idiopathic and neurogenic bladder overactivity populations, respectively. These results suggest that BoNT-A may be a more durable treatment for detrusor overactivity.

Bladder injection technique

In earlier series, bladder injections of BoNT were performed with a rigid cystoscope under spinal or general anesthesia. Currently, less invasive techniques with a flexible cystoscope under local anesthesia are popular [29]. Patients are treated in an outpatient setting after local anesthetization with intraurethral 2% lidocaine jelly and 30 mL of intravesical 2% lidocaine for 10 minutes (Fig. 1). Using a 25-gauge flexible, disposable injection needle (Olympus, Melville, New York) inserted through a flexible cystoscope, 200 U of BoNT-A diluted in 20 mL of preservative-free saline is injected submucosally into 20 sites within the bladder trigone and base. All patients receive perioperative oral antibiotics and are followed up subjectively by phone or by office interview

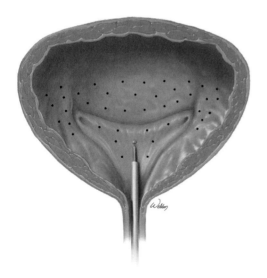

Fig. 1. Injection technique for BoNT into the overactive bladder.

in addition to postvoid residual measurement with bladder ultrasound during clinic visits.

Science and mechanism of action of botulinum toxin

Efferent cholinergic effect

Clinical success with intradetrusor BoNT injections is supported by basic science research demonstrating the efficacy of BoNT on autonomic nerves (Box 1). Smith and colleagues [35] found significant decreases in the release of labeled acetylcholine in BoNT-A–injected normal rat bladders after high but not low frequency stimulation. Somogyi and co-investigators [36] previously showed that presynaptic muscarinic facilitatory mechanisms are upregulated in cholinergic nerve terminals of SCI bladders, leading to a larger relative contractile response at lower frequencies of stimulation. Thus, although a significant inhibitory effect of BoNT-A on acetylcholine release at low frequencies of stimulation was not demonstrated in normal rat bladders, one could hypothesize that such an effect might occur in SCI rat bladders. If similar relationships exist in human bladders, then BoNT-A may be an effective treatment for uninhibited nonvoiding contractions characteristic of all forms of detrusor overactivity.

Afferent cholinergic effect

The efficacy of BoNT-A in conditions of detrusor overactivity may result from an inhibitory effect on detrusor muscle. Some effects of the drug may also be mediated by altering afferent (sensory) input. Urothelium possesses muscarinic receptor populations with a density two times that of detrusor smooth muscle, and dorsal root ganglionectomy experiments demonstrating the persistence of acetylcholinesterase-staining nerves near the urothelium suggest that parasympathetic nerves supply some innervation to urothelium [37–39]. In addition to receiving cholinergic innervation, human urothelium has also been shown to release the neurotransmitter acetylcholine at rest [40]. Thus, acetylcholine, released from urothelium and acting on nearby muscarinic receptor populations (ie, urothelium or afferent nerves) or neuronal sources of acetylcholine binding to muscarinic receptors within urothelium or afferent nerves, could have a significant impact on bladder sensory input to the central nervous system and may be impacted by BoNT treatment (Fig. 2).

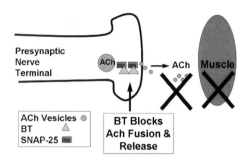

Fig. 2. Hypothesized antinociceptive effects of BoNT on the bladder. ACh, acetylcholine; BT, botulinum toxin.

Inhibition of ATP release

The inhibitory effect of BoNT on detrusor overactivity is not limited to its effects on acetylcholine release. For example, contractile data suggest that BoNT-A may impair ATP release in addition to acetylcholine release from isolated bladder tissue [41]. These results have clinical significance in lieu of recent investigations of alterations in P2X receptor expression and increased purinergic bladder response in patients who have idiopathic detrusor instability. O'Reilly and colleagues [42] found that approximately 50% of the nerve-mediated contractions in bladder tissues extracted from patients who had IDO were purinergic in origin.

In addition, recent basic and clinical evidence suggests that BoNT-A may have antinociceptive effects unrelated to its actions on efferent nerve terminals [43–45]. By impairing urothelial or afferent nerve transmitter release, particularly under conditions of chronic inflammation or SCI, BoNT-A could reduce peripheral sensitization mechanisms that are thought to play an important role in increasing afferent nerve activity. An in vitro model of mechanoreceptor-stimulated urothelial ATP release was tested in SCI rat bladders to determine whether intravesical BoNT-A administration would inhibit urothelial ATP release, a measure of sensory nerve activation [46]. The results demonstrated that hypo-osmotic stimulation of bladder urothelium evokes a significant release of ATP that is markedly inhibited (53%) by BoNT-A, suggesting that impairment of urothelial ATP release may be one mechanism by which BoNT-A reduces detrusor overactivity.

Summary

BoNT has proved to be a safe and effective therapy for a variety of autonomic motor disorders. Urologists are now finding clinical success

with bladder BoNT-A injections in the treatment of neurogenic and IDO. It is important to remember that the application of BoNT in the lower urinary tract is not approved by the regulatory agencies and caution should be applied until larger randomized clinical studies are completed.

References

[1] Erbguth FJ. Historical notes on botulism, *Clostridium botulinum*, botulinum toxin, and the idea of the therapeutic use of the toxin. Mov Disord 2004; 19(8):S2–6.

[2] Petit H, Wiart E, Gaujard E, et al. Botulinum A toxin treatment for detrusor-sphincter dyssynergia in spinal cord disease. Spinal Cord 1998;36(2):91–4.

[3] Dykstra DD, Sidi A. Treatment of detrusor-sphincter dyssynergia with botulinum A toxin: a double blind study. Arch Phys Med Rehabil 1990;71(1):24–6.

[4] Dykstra DD, Sidi AA, Scott AB, et al. Effects of botulinum A toxin on detrusor-sphincter dyssyngeria in spinal cord injury patients. J Urol 1988;139(5): 919–22.

[5] Chancellor MB, de Groat WC. Intravesical capsaicin and resiniferatoxin: spicing up the ways to treat the overactive bladder. J Urol 1999;162(1):3–11.

[6] Stohrer M, Schurch B, Kramer G, et al. Botulinum A-toxin in the treatment of detrusor hyperreflexia in spinal cord injured patients: a new alternative to medical and surgical procedures? Neurourol Urodyn 1999;18(4):401.

[7] Schurch B, Stohrer M, Kramer G, et al. Botulinum-A toxin for treating detrusor hyperreflexia in spinal cord injured patients: a new alternative to anticholinergic drugs? Preliminary results. J Urol 2000;164: 692–7.

[8] Del Popolo G. Botulinum-A toxin in the treatment of detrusor hyperreflexia [abstract]. Neurourol Urodyn 2001;20(4):522–4.

[9] Heckmann M, Ceballos-Baumann AO, Plewig G. Hyperhidrosis study group: botulinum toxin A for axillary hyperhidrosis (excessive sweating). N Engl J Med 2001;344(7):488–93.

[10] Porta M, Gamba M, Bertacchi G, et al. Treatment of sialorrhoea with ultrasound guided botulinum toxin type A injection in patients with neurological disorders. J Neurol Neurosurg Psychiatry 2001;70(4): 538–40.

[11] Von Lindern JJ, Niederhagen B, Berge S, et al. Frey syndrome: treatment with type A botulinum toxin. Cancer 2000;89(8):1659–63.

[12] Schurch B, Stöhrer M, Kramer G, et al. Botulinum toxin-A to treat detrusor hyperreflexia in spinal cord injured patients [abstract]. Neurourol Urodyn 2001;20(4):521–2.

[13] Reitz A, Stohrer M, Kramer G, et al. European experience of 200 cases treated with botulinum-A toxin injections into the detrusor muscle for urinary

incontinence due to neurogenic detrusor overactivity. Eur Urol 2004;45:510–5.

[14] Klaphajone J, Kitisomprayoonkul W, Sriplakit S. Botulinum toxin type A for treating neurogenic detrusor overactivty combined with low-compliance bladder in patients with spinal cord lesions. Arch Phys Med Rehabil 2005;86:2114–8.

[15] Schurch B, de Seze M, Denys P, et al. Botulinum-A toxin type A is a safe and effective treatment for neurogenic urinary incontinence: results of a single treatment, randomized, placebo controlled 6-month study. J Urol 2005;174:196–200.

[16] Schulte-Baukloh H, Michael T, Sturzebecher B, et al. Botulinum A-toxin detrusor injection as a novel approach in the treatment of bladder spasticity in children with neurogenic bladder. Eur Urol 2003; 44:139–43.

[17] Riccabona M, Koen M, Schindler M, et al. Botulinum-A toxin injection into the detrusor: a safe alternative in the treatment of children with myelomeningocele with detrusor hyperreflexia. J Urol 2004;171:845–8.

[18] Giannantoni A, Di Stasi SM, Stephen RL, et al. Intravesical resiniferatoxin versus botulinum-A toxin injections for neurogenic detrusor overactivity: a prospective randomized study. J Urol 2004;172:240–3.

[19] de Paiva A, Meunier FA, Molgo J, et al. Functional repair of motor endplates after botulinum neurotoxin type A poisoning: biphasic switch of synaptic activity between nerve sprouts and their parent terminals. Proc Natl Acad Sci U S A 1999;96(6):3200–5.

[20] Greene P, Fahn S, Diamond B. Development of resistance to botulinum toxin type A in patients with torticollis. Mov Disord 1994;9(2):213–7.

[21] Jankovic J, Vuong KD, Ahsan J. Comparison of efficacy and immunogenicity of original versus current botulinum toxin in cervical dystonia. Neurology 2003;60(7):1186–8.

[22] Whelchel DD, Brehmer TM, Brooks PM, et al. Molecular targets of botulinum toxin at the mammalian neuromuscular junction. Mov Disord 2004;19(Suppl 8):S7–16.

[23] Haferkamp A, Schurch B, Reitz A, et al. Lack of ultrastructural detrusor changes following endoscopic injection of botulinum toxin type A in overactive neurogenic bladder. Eur Urol 2004;46(6):784–91.

[24] Grosse JO, Kramer G, Lochner-Ernst D, et al. Outcome of repeat detrusor injections of botulinum A toxin (BTX-A) for severe neurogenic detrusor overactivity and incontinence. J Urol 2003;169 (4 Suppl):373.

[25] Schulte-Baukloh H, Knispel HH, Stolze T, et al. Repeated botulinum-A toxin injections in treatment of children with neurogenic detrusor overactivity. Urology 2005;66(4):865–70 [discussion: 870].

[26] Radziszewski P, Dobronski P, Borkowski A. Treatment of the non-neurogenic storage and voiding

disorders with the chemical denervation caused by botulinum toxin type A—a pilot study [abstract]. Neurourol Urodyn 2001;20(4):410–2.

[27] Zermann DH, Ishigooka M, Schubert J, et al. Trigonum and bladder base injection of botulinum toxin A (BTX) in patients with severe urgency-frequency-syndrome refractory to conservative medical treatment and electrical stimulation [abstract]. Neurourol Urodyn 2001;20(4):412–3.

[28] Loch A, Loch T, Osterhage J, et al. Botulinum-A toxin detrusor injections in the treatment of non-neurologic and neurologic cases of urge incontinence. J Urol 2003;169(4 Suppl):124.

[29] Smith CP, Nishiguchi J, O'Leary M, et al. Single institution experience in 110 patients with botulinum toxin-A injection into the bladder or urethra. Urology 2005;65:37–41.

[30] Rapp DE, Lucioni A, Katz EE, et al. Use of botulinum-A toxin for the treatment of refractory overactive bladder symptoms: an initial experience. Urology 2004;63:1071–5.

[31] Werner M, Schmid DM, Schussler B. Efficacy of botulinum-A toxin in the treatment of detrusor overactivity incontinence: a prospective nonrandomized study. Am J Obstet Gynecol 2005;192(5):1735–40.

[32] Kessler TM, Danuser H, Schumacher M, et al. Botulinum A toxin injections into the detrusor: an effective treatment in idiopathic and neurogenic detrusor overactivity? Neurourol Urodyn 2005;24(3):231–6.

[33] Popat R, Apostolidis A, Kalsi V, et al. A comparison between the response of patients with idiopathic detrusor overactivity and neurogenic detrusor overactivity to the first intradetrusor injection of botulinum-A toxin. J Urol 2005;174(3):984–9.

[34] Dykstra D, Enriquez A, Valley M. Treatment of overactive bladder with botulinum toxin type B: a pilot study. Int Urogynecol J 2003;14:424–6.

[35] Smith CP, Franks ME, McNeil BK, et al. Effect of botulinum toxin A on the autonomic nervous system of the rat lower urinary tract. J Urol 2003;169(5):1896–900.

[36] Somogyi GT, Zernova GV, Yoshiyama M, et al. Frequency dependence of muscarinic facilitation of transmitter release in urinary bladder strips from neurally intact or chronic spinal cord transected rats. Br J Pharmacol 1998;125(2):241–6.

[37] Hawthorn MH, Chapple CR, Cock M, et al. Urothelium-derived inhibitory factor(s) influence detrusor muscle contractility in vitro. Br J Pharmacol 2000;129:416–9.

[38] Wakabayashi Y, Kojima Y, Makiura Y, et al. Free terminal fibers of autonomic nerves in the mucosa of the cat urinary bladder. In: Wegmann RJ, Wegmann MA, editors. Recent advances in cellular and molecular biology, vol. 3. Leuven, Belgium: Peeters Press; 1991. p. 109–17.

[39] Wakabayashi Y, Kojima Y, Makiura Y, et al. Acetyl-cholinesterase positive axons in the mucosa of urinary bladder of adult cats: retrograde tracing and degeneration studies. Histol Histopathol 1995;10:523–30.

[40] Andersson KE, Yoshida M. Antimuscarinics and the overactive detrusor—which is the main mechanism of action? Eur Urol 2003;43(1):1–5.

[41] Smith CP, Boone TB, de Groat WC, et al. Effect of stimulation intensity and botulinum toxin isoform on rat bladder strip contractions. Brain Res Bull 2003;61:165–71.

[42] O'Reilly BA, Kosaka AH, Knight GF, et al. P2X receptors and their role in female idiopathic detrusor instability. J Urol 2002;167:157–64.

[43] Cui M, Khanijou S, Rubino J, et al. Subcutaneous administration of botulinum toxin A reduces formalin-induced pain. Pain 2004;107(1–2):125–33.

[44] Vemulakonda VM, Somogyi GT, Kiss S, et al. Inhibitory effect of intravesically applied botulinum toxin A in chronic bladder inflammation. J Urol 2005;173(2):621–4.

[45] Smith CP, Chancellor MB. Emerging role of botulinum toxin in the management of voiding dysfunction. J Urol 2004;171:2128–37.

[46] Khera M, Somogyi GT, Kiss S, et al. Botulinum toxin A inhibits ATP release from bladder urothelium after chronic spinal cord injury. Neurochem Int 2004;45:987–93.

ELSEVIER
SAUNDERS

Urol Clin N Am 33 (2006) 511–518

Local Effects of Antimuscarinics

Hitoshi Masuda, MD, PhD[a], Yong-Tae Kim, MD, PhD[b],
Shachi Tyagi, MD[c], Michael B. Chancellor, MD[c],
Fernando de Miguel, PhD[c], Naoki Yoshimura, MD, PhD[c],*

[a]*Department of Urology and Reproductive Medicine, Graduate School,
Tokyo Medical and Dental University, Tokyo, Japan*
[b]*Department of Urology, College of Medicine, Hanyang University,
Seoul, South Korea*
[c]*Department of Urology, University of Pittsburgh School of Medicine, Kaufmann Medical Building,
Suite 700, 3471 Fifth Avenue, Pittsburgh, PA 15213-3221, USA*

Overactive bladder (OAB) syndrome, clinically characterized by symptoms of urgency usually associated with frequency and nocturia, with or without urge incontinence [1], has been estimated to occur in nearly 17% of the population, and the syndrome increases with age [2]. The most common drug treatments for OAB are antimuscarinic agents [3]. These agents clinically act to increase bladder capacity and to decrease the urge to urinate during the storage phase when there is normally no activity in parasympathetic nerves [4]. Evaluations of efficacy of antimuscarinic agents, however, have traditionally been based on the inhibitory effects of detrusor muscle contractions, mainly through suppression of the muscarinic receptor subtype M_3 [3,5–7]. Thus, recently, an increasing number of studies have focused on the role and mechanism of muscarinic acetylcholine receptors (mAChRs) for the regulation of afferent activity during urine storage [8].

The urothelium has been considered a simple inert barrier; however, it is metabolically active, and recent studies have reported that the urothelium acts as an important regulator of bladder contractility or sensation [9,10]. It has also been

reported that mAChRs are located on the urothelium [11–13] and that basal release of acetylcholine (ACh) from the urothelium increases with age and stretch [14]. In the case of OAB, release of ACh during the urine storage phase may be an important contributor to its pathophysiology [15,16]. Therefore, there are possibilities that (1) non-neuronal ACh released from the urothelium can activate mAChRs, leading to modulation of afferent pathways during the micturition reflex, and (2) increased ACh levels in the bladder can induce OAB mediated by the local effects on mAChRs. Thus, muscarinic receptor–mediated bladder sensory mechanisms may represent an additional site of action of the muscarinic receptor antagonists (antimuscarinics) that are used for the treatment of OAB.

Muscarinic receptors in the bladder urothelium

Radioligand-binding studies with [³H] quinuclidinyl benzylate have indicated that in humans, the density of mAChRs in the bladder mucosa was equal to that in the detrusor [17], whereas in the pig, the density of mAChRs in the mucosa was higher than that in the detrusor [11]. Immunohistochemical staining of human bladder tissues with an antibody directed against choline acetyltransferase detected the presence of immunoreactive cells in smooth muscles and urothelium. The immunoreactivity in the urothelium was relatively higher in elderly patients than in younger patients

This work was supported by grants from the National Institutes of Health (DK57267, DK68557, DK66138, P01 HD39768) and Indevus, Inc.

* Corresponding author.

E-mail address: nyos@pitt.edu (N. Yoshimura).

[14]. Overall, these findings indicate the presence of cholinergic mechanisms in the urothelium.

Muscarinic receptor subtypes in the detrusor and urothelium

Five subtypes of G protein–coupled mAChRs (M_1–M_5) have been cloned and pharmacologically characterized. Detrusor smooth muscle from several species contains M_2 and M_3 receptor subtypes [5,9,18]. The ratio of M_2 to M_3 in the bladder is 9:1 in the rat but 3:1 in other species [18]. In the human bladder, the occurrence of mRNA for all mAChR subtypes has been demonstrated, with a predominant expression of mRNA encoding M_2 and M_3 receptors [19,20]. Recently, competitive-binding assay experiments in humans indicated receptor populations of 71% M_2, 22% M_3, and 7% M_1 in the detrusor muscle and 75% M_2 and 25% M_3/M_5 in the mucosa (urothelium and suburothelium). In addition, using reverse transcriptase polymerase chain reaction (RT-PCR), expression of M_1, M_2, M_3, and M_5 mRNA was demonstrated in detrusor and in mucosa. The detrusor and the mucosa did not show any visible expression of M_4 receptor mRNA with RT-PCR [17]. Recently, Tyagi and colleagues [12] also reported the presence of mRNA coding for M_1, M_2, M_3, and M_4 not only in fresh bladder tissues but also in primary cultures of urothelial cells and detrusor muscles of the human bladder.

Immunohistochemical studies have also suggested that in the rat, M_1, M_2, M_3, M_4, and M_5 mAChRs were present in the urothelium [13]. The extent of expression of the urothelial muscarinic receptors, however, seems to vary substantially depending on pathologic conditions because in cyclophosphamide-pretreated rat bladders, there was a dramatic increase in the immunoreactivity of M_5 receptors [13].

Non-neuronal acetylcholine

It is well known that postganglionic parasympathetic neurons are the major source of ACh in the bladder; however, it has been reported that non-neuronal ACh is synthesized in cells other than neurons and may act in an autocrine or paracrine manner [21,22]. Non-neuronal ACh has also been detected in bronchial and placental epithelial cells, the mucosa of alimentary tract, the corneal epithelium, keratinocytes, glandular tissues, endothelial cells, and blood cells [21–24].

In the human bladder, functional and microdialysis experiments indicate that cholinergic nerve-mediated bladder contractions and neuronal ACh released by electrical field stimulation are decreased with age, suggesting that neurogenic cholinergic transmission is reduced with age [14]. Radioligand-binding studies also indicated a decrease in total muscarinic receptors in the bladder with age. Moreover, RT-PCR methods showed a decrease in the level of expression of M_3 receptor mRNA with age but no corresponding changes in M_2 receptor mRNA of human bladders [17]. In contrast, non-neuronal ACh has been reported to increase with age [14]. In addition, non-neuronal ACh from the urothelium has been reported to increase with bladder stretch [14]. Thus, these results suggest that ACh released from the urothelium may be a factor contributing to mechanoafferent transduction to modulate the micturition reflex and that increased expression of non-neuronal ACh could contribute to the emergence of OAB symptoms and detrusor overactivity.

Acetylcholine and muscarinic acetylcholine receptors related to functional modulation of afferent pathways

Recent data suggest that bladder stretch or small contractions can cause the release of different factors from the urothelium, including ATP, prostaglandins [10,25,26], and nitric oxide [27]. It is generally thought that ATP and prostaglandins can stimulate afferent neurons [10,25,26], whereas nitric oxide can inhibit afferent activity [27]. Therefore, it is possible that non-neuronal ACh released from the urothelium by distension and small contractions of the detrusor can also activate mAChRs located on afferent nerve endings in the suburothelial layer to induce detrusor overactivity. If this theory is true, then non-neuronal ACh release in the storage phase of the micturition reflex may help to explain the effectiveness of antimuscarinic agents for the treatment of OAB caused by detrusor overactivity. As far as the authors know, there is no direct confirmation about the existence of mAChRs located on afferent fibers in the suburothelial layer; however, RT-PCR has revealed that M_2, M_3, and M_5 but not M_1 or M_4 mAChR subtypes are expressed in L6 and S1 dorsal root ganglions (DRGs). These

DRGs contain most of the bladder afferent neurons sending their axons in the pelvic nerve. It has also been shown by using patch clamp recordings that mAChR activation exhibits excitatory and inhibitory effects in different types of afferent neurons from lumbosacral DRGs [28,29]. Taken together, these findings suggest that ACh may stimulate mAChRs located on afferent fibers, leading to detrusor overactivity. Activation of mAChRs in primary cultured rat urothelial cells using ACh can reportedly release two transmitters (nitric oxide and ATP) [28], suggesting that local increases in ACh may stimulate urothelial mAChRs, leading to modulation of ATP release that can also induce detrusor overactivity by activation of purinergic P2X receptors located on afferent nerves [30].

In other fields, muscarine or arecaidine (mAChR agonists) induced inhibition of capsaicin-evoked calcitonin gene-related peptide (CGRP) release from buccal mucosa in a gallamine (an M_2 receptor antagonist)-sensitive manner, indicating that M_2 mAChR activation leads to a decrease in peripheral nociceptor activity. In addition, investigations on C-nociceptors in the skin-nerve preparation have demonstrated that arecaidine caused a significant, concentration-dependent decrease in noxious heat-evoked CGRP release and that M_2 mAChRs exert an inhibitory or desensitizing influence on the peripheral terminals of C-nociceptors [31,32]. In situ hybridization also demonstrated that M_2 mRNA was present in trigeminal ganglion neurons and coexpressed with CGRP or TRPV1 capsaicin receptor [30]. Thus, M_2 receptors in primary afferent pathways may represent a viable peripheral target for the treatment of pain and inflammation.

Functional studies related to bladder muscarinic acetylcholine receptors

It has been reported that M_3 knockout mice of either sex had longer voiding intervals and increased micturition volumes than wild-type controls, suggesting that muscarinic receptors, especially M_3 receptors, may be involved in volume threshold regulation for micturition during the storage phase [33].

Recently, the authors reported that intravesical application of carbachol or ACh can induce detrusor overactivity in rats. Because intravesical application of mAChRs agonists such as oxotremoline-M or arecaidine similarly induced detrusor overactivity, excitation of local mAChRs in the bladder is likely to be responsible for detrusor overactivity induced by intravesical carbachol or ACh [34,35]. In addition, subcutaneous capsaicin pretreatment (125 mg/kg, 4 days before the experiments) did not prevent ACh-, oxotremoline-M –, or arecaidine-induced detrusor overactivity (Fig. 1) [35], whereas ATP-induced detrusor overactivity has been reported to be suppressed by capsaicin pretreatment [30]. These findings suggest that muscarinic but not purinergic excitatory effects on afferent pathways in the bladder are mediated by way of capsaicin-resistant bladder afferent pathways.

It has been suggested that bladder phasic activity during the filling phase may have a role in generating or modulating afferent discharge in sensory nerves, thereby providing a mechanism capable of affecting bladder sensations [36,37]. Recently, phasic rises in intravesical pressure were reported to be generated by a network of interstitial cells or myofibroblasts within the suburothelial layer [36,38,39]. These cells have some of the structural characteristics of smooth muscles and of fibroblasts. These cells also express M_3 mAChRs [36] and are associated with diffuse innervation of large myelinated and small unmyelinated fibers including A delta and C fibers, [38,39], a feature similarly observed with myofibroblasts in other tissues [40]. These findings have postulated a potential role of suburothelial myofibroblasts in the sensation of bladder fullness [39,41]. Thus, myofibroblasts are in an ideal position, interposed between the urothelium and nerve endings, to form an intermediary layer in the sensory process. Therefore, exogenous and endogenous ACh might stimulate suburothelial interstitial cells such as myofibroblasts, leading to stimulation of capsaicin-resistant afferent pathways rather than direct stimulation of afferent nerves. Although this assumption seems reasonable, functional interactions between myofibroblasts and ACh should be further clarified in future studies.

It has also been reported that intravesical application of carbachol enhanced spinal ATP release in normal and chronic spinal cord–injured rats and that spinal cord injury induced a dramatic increase in basal and stimulated ATP release in the spinal cord, suggesting that a spinal ATP pathway might be involved during excitation of mAChRs in the bladder to induce detrusor overactivity [42].

Another important issue is that urothelial muscarinic mechanisms may have not only

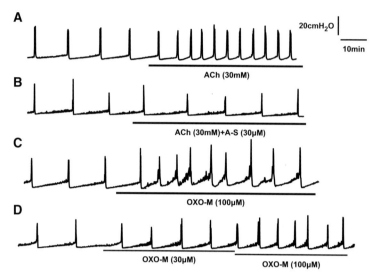

Fig. 1. Typical cystometric findings in urethane anesthetized rats. (*A*) Intercontraction intervals (ICI) were decreased with intravesical application of Ach (30 mM). (*B*) Effects of intravesical injection of atropine sulfate (A-S, 30 μM) on ACh (30 mM)-induced bladder activity. (*C*) ICI was decreased with intravesical oxotremoline-M (OXO-M, 100 μM). (*D*) Capsaicin pretreatment did not prevent intravesical OXO-M–induced bladder activity. Bars indicate the timing for applying the compound.

excitatory but also inhibitory effects on afferent activity. Recent studies in pig and human bladder strips have suggested that activation of urothelial mAChRs by carbachol resulted in the release of an inhibitory factor that can reduce detrusor contractility [11,43]. In addition, activation of mAChRs in primary cultured rat urothelial cells by ACh has been reported to release the excitatory and inhibitory transmitters ATP and nitric oxide, respectively [28]. Therefore, in the normal state, autoregulatory mechanisms may exist in urothelial muscarinic receptor function.

Antimuscarinic agents

It has been reported that in anesthetized rats that had acetone-induced cystitis, high-dose oxybutynin but not atropine prolonged micturition intervals and significantly suppressed micturition pressure, suggesting that the effects of oxybutynin on micturition intervals are considered to be mainly linked to its direct smooth muscle–relaxant effect [44,45]. Oxybutynin was also shown to increase micturition intervals in spinal cord–injured rats, although the systemic effective dose for increasing micturition intervals seemed to be higher than the dose affecting bladder contractions [46]. Antimuscarinics at clinically recommended doses,

however, have little effect on voiding contractions and may act mainly during the bladder storage phase. Sasaki and colleagues [47] reported no effects of oxybutynin (intraduodenal) on bladder capacity in sham-operated and nerve-transected rats. It was also demonstrated that systemic administration of oxybutynin and tolterodine did not prevent a decrease in micturition intervals caused by intravesical acetic acid, although it decreased micturition voiding pressure in rats [48]. Capsaicin pretreatment has been reported to significantly suppress acetic acid–induced detrusor overactivity [49] but failed to affect mAChR-mediated detrusor overactivity [35]. Therefore, inhibition of mAChRs in the bladder may have no effect on detrusor overactivity mediated by activation of capsaicin-sensitive C-fiber afferents.

Oxybutynin has been shown to have antimuscarinic and so-called "direct muscle–relaxant" or "local anesthetic" actions [50]. In vitro, however, oxybutynin is 500 times weaker as a smooth muscle relaxant than it is as an antimuscarinic agent [51]. Therefore, when given systemically at doses used clinically, oxybutynin acts mainly as an antimuscarinic drug, whereas direct effects may be of importance when the drug is administered intravesically. Intravesical oxybutynin has proved to be clinically effective for the treatment of detrusor overactivity and, therefore, it is used in OAB patients who are refractory to oral administration or cannot tolerate the oral medication [52,53]. Previous experiments indicated that intravesical oxybutynin has a direct anesthetic effect within the bladder wall by temporarily desensitizing C-fiber afferents without affecting A delta fibers, which could explain its clinical benefits for OAB treatment [54]. Intravesical and intravenous tolterodine was also reported to improve detrusor overactivity mediated by way of suppression of C-fiber bladder afferent nerves [55]. Tolterodine also demonstrated an antagonistic effect on neurokinin-2 receptors [56]; thus, inhibitory effects of tolterodine on C-fiber afferent pathways might be attributable to suppression of neurokinin-2 receptors in C-fiber bladder afferents [55].

Recently, it was reported that the antimuscarinic agents oxybutynin and tolterodine but not atropine or trospium are capable of significantly modulating L-, N-, and P/Q-type high-voltage calcium channel activity of DRG neurons innervating the urinary bladder. Functionally, oxybutinin and tolterodine are reportedly modulators of L-type calcium channels. These findings suggest that oxybutynin and tolterodine may exert direct effects on bladder sensory pathways through modulation of calcium channels in addition to antimuscarinic activity [57].

The authors recently reported that intravesical application of carbachol-induced detrusor overactivity was prevented by concomitant application of oxybutynin, trospium, tolterodine, or dimethindene (an M_2-selective mAChR antagonist) without affecting bladder contraction pressure. These results suggest that M_2-muscarinic receptors are involved in the emergence of bladder overactivity in situations in which there is high ACh release in the bladder [34]. It has also been reported that the M_2 receptor antagonist methoctramine significantly increased the voiding interval and bladder compliance in rats that had acetic acid–induced detrusor overactivity, and significantly reduced the number of spontaneous contractions in a rat model of bladder outlet obstruction [58]. It is known that M_2 receptor activation can oppose sympathetically mediated detrusor relaxation by way of β-adrenoceptors because activation of M_2 receptors results in inhibition of adenylyl cyclase [59]. Therefore, M_2 receptors in the urothelium, bladder afferent pathways, or myofibroblasts might be a potential target for the treatment of OAB, although further studies are needed to clarify this point.

The authors reported that intravesically applied ACh-induced detrusor overactivity was prevented not only by concomitant application of atropine but also by intravenous application of atropine, oxybutynin, trospium, and tolterodine dose dependently [35]. Recently, the authors also demonstrated that urine excreted after oral ingestion of trospium had a significant inhibitory effect in a rat model of detrusor overactivity induced by intravesical carbachol [60]. In this study, two "normal" adult volunteers collected voided urine after taking trospium, tolterodine (once a day formula), or oxybutynin (once a day formula). Next, the effect of intravesical administration of human urine on carbachol-induced bladder overactivity was studied in rats. Although human urine, with or without intake of antimuscarinic agents, had no effect on normal bladder function, urine collected from the volunteers who had taken trospium but not tolterodine or oxybutynin prevented the carbachol-induced reduction in bladder capacity and intercontraction intervals [60]. These results suggest that antimuscarinic agents such as trospium, which are excreted into urine with active metabolites in a significant fraction [61], might be more effective for treating detrusor overactivity because of their local effect in addition to the systemic effects on mAChRs in bladder smooth muscles.

Until now, very few studies have examined whether ACh release and expression of mAChRs in the urothelium or suburothelium can change in different pathologic conditions such as inflammation, bladder outlet obstruction, spinal cord injury, and so forth, which result in detrusor overactivity. Further investigations should be performed to clarify the roles of local muscarinic–afferent interaction mechanisms in the control of lower urinary tract function.

Summary

It is likely that local muscarinic receptors have an important role in the modulation of bladder afferent excitability and voiding. Thus, interactions between muscarinic receptors in the urothelium, afferent nerves, or myofibroblasts and locally released ACh that is increased by bladder stretch and aging might be involved in the emergence of detrusor overactivity and OAB (see Fig. 2). Therefore, antimuscarinic agents may be effective in treating OAB not only by suppression of muscarinic receptor–mediated detrusor muscle contractions but also by modulation of muscarinic receptor–bladder afferent interactions.

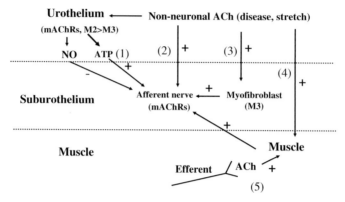

Fig. 2. Possible mechanisms for muscarinic receptor-mediated sensory function of non-neuronal ACh. (*1*) Activation of afferent nerves mediated by way of urothelium-derived ATP. (*2*) Direct activation of afferent nerves. (*3*) Activation of afferent nerves by way of excitation of myofibroblasts. (*4*) Activation of afferent nerves by way of excitation of muscles (enhancement of myogenic activity). Tonic release of ACh from afferent nerves. (*5*) Activation of afferent nerves by way of excitation of muscles (enhancement of myogenic activity). NO, nitric oxide.

References

[1] Abrams P, Cardozo L, Fall M, et al. The standardisation of terminology of lower urinary tract function: report from the Standardisation Sub-Committee of the International Continence Society. Neurourol Urodyn 2002;21:167–78.

[2] Milsom I, Abrams P, Cardozo L, et al. How widespread are the symptoms of an overactive bladder and how are they managed? A population-based prevalence study. BJU Int 2001;87:760–6.

[3] Yamanishi T, Chapple CR, Chess-Williams R. Which muscarinic receptor is important in the bladder? World J Urol 2001;19:299–306.

[4] De Groat WC, Booth AM, Yoshimura N. Neurophysiology of micturition and its modifications in animal models of human disease. In: Maggi CA, editor. The autonomic nervous system nervous control of the urogenital system, vol. 6. London: Harwood; 1993. p. 227–89.

[5] Hegde SS, Eglen RM. Muscarinic receptor subtypes modulating smooth muscle contractility in the urinary bladder. Life Sci 1999;64:419–28.

[6] Chess-Williams R, Chapple CR, Yamanishi T, et al. The minor population of M3-receptors mediate contraction of human detrusor muscle in vitro. J Auton Pharmacol 2001;21:243–8.

[7] Fetscher C, Fleichman M, Schmidt M, et al. M(3) muscarinic receptors mediate contraction of human urinary bladder. Br J Pharmacol 2002;136:641–3.

[8] Andersson K-E, Yoshida M. Antimuscarinic and the overactive detrusor—which is the main mechanism of action? Eur Urol 2003;43:1–5.

[9] Chess-Williams R. Muscarinic receptors of the urinary bladder: detrusor, urothelial and prejunctional. Auton Autocoid Pharmacol 2002;22:133–45.

[10] Fry CH, Ikeda Y, Harvey R, et al. Control of bladder function by peripheral nerves: avenues for novel drug targets. Urology 2004;63(Suppl 1):24–31.

[11] Hawthorn MH, Chapple CR, Cock M, et al. Urothelium-derived inhibitory factor(s) influences on detrusor muscle contractility in vitro. Br J Pharmacol 2000;129:416–9.

[12] Tyagi S, Le TSV, Thomas CA, et al. Differentiation stage-specific expression patterns of muscarinic receptors 1–5 mRNA in urothelium and detrusor of human bladder. J Urol 2005;173:325.

[13] Giglio D, Ryberg AT, To K, et al. Altered muscarinic receptor subtype and functional responses in cyclophosphamide induced cyctitis in rats. Auton Neurosci Basic Clin 2005;122:9–20.

[14] Yoshida M, Miyamae K, Iwashita H, et al. Management of detrusor dysfunction in the elderly: changes in acetylcholine and adenosine triphosphate release during aging. Urology 2004;63:17–23.

[15] Smith PH, Cook JB, Prasad EW. The effect of ubretid on bladder function after recent complete spinal cord injury. Br J Urol 1974;46:187–92.

[16] Yossepowitch O, Gillon G, Baniel J, et al. The effect of cholinergic enhancement during filling cystometry: can edrophonium chloride be used as a provocative test for overactive bladder? J Urol 2001;165:1441–5.

[17] Mansfield KJ, Liu L, Mitchelson FJ, et al. Muscarnic receptor subtypes in human bladder and mucosa, studied by radioligand binding and quantitative competitive RT-PCR: changes in ageing. Br J Pharmacol 2005;144:1089–99.

[18] Wang P, Luthin GR, Ruggieri MR. Muscarinic acetylcholine receptor subtypes mediating urinary bladder contractility and coupling to GTP binding proteins. J Pharmacol Exp Ther 1995;273:959–66.

[19] Sigala S, Mirabella G, Peroni A, et al. Differential gene expression of cholinergic muscarinic receptor subtypes in male and female normal human urinary bladder. Urology 2002;60:719–25.

[20] Yamaguchi O, Shishido K, Tamura K, et al. Evaluation of mRNAs encoding muscarinic receptor subtypes in human detrusor muscle. J Urol 1996;156:1208–13.

[21] Wessler I, Krikpatrick CJ, Rache K. Non-neuronal acetylcholine a locally acting molecule, widely distributed in biological systems: expression and function in humans. Pharmacol Ther 1998;77:59–79.

[22] Klapproth H, Reinheimer T, Metzen J, et al. Non-neuronal acetylcholine, a signalling molecule synthesized by surface cells of rat and man. Naunyn Schmiedebergs Arch Pharmacol 1997;355:513–23.

[23] Sastry BV. Human placental cholinergic system. Biochem Pharmacol 1997;53:1577–86.

[24] Conti-Fine BM, Navaneetham D, Lei S, et al. Neuronal nicotinic receptors in non-neural cells: new mediators of tobacco toxicity? Eur J Pharmacol 2000;393:279–94.

[25] de Groat WC. The urothelium in overactive bladder: passive bystander or active participant? Urology 2004;64:7–11.

[26] Maggi CA. Prostanoids as local modulators of reflex micturition. Pharmacol Res 1992;25:13–20.

[27] Yoshimura N, Seki S, Chancellor MB, et al. Targeting afferent hyperexcitability for therapy of the painful bladder syndrome. Urology 2002;59:61–7.

[28] Beckel JM, Barrick SR, Keast JR, et al. Expression and function of urothelial muscarinic receptors and interactions with bladder nerves. Abstr Soc Neurosci 2004;846.

[29] Negoita FA, Beckel JM, Birder LA, et al. Effects of muscarinic receptor agonists on lumbosacral dorsal root ganglion cells. Abstr Soc Neurosci 2004;950.

[30] Nishiguchi J, Hayashi Y, Chancellor MB, et al. Detrusor overactivity induced by intravesical application of adenosine of adenosine 5'-triphosphate under different delivery conditions in rats. Urology 2005;66:1332–7.

[31] Dussor GO, Helesic G, Hargreaves KM, et al. Cholinergic modulation of nociceptive responses in vivo and neuropeptide release in vitro at the level of the primary sensory neurons. Pain 2004;107:22–32.

[32] Bernardini N, Roza C, Sauer SK, et al. Muscarinic M2 receptors on peripheral nerve endings: a molecular target of antinociception. J Neurosci 2002;22:1–5.

[33] Igawa W, Zhang X, Nishizawa O, et al. Cystometric findings in mice lacking muscarinic M2 or M3 receptors. J Urol 2004;172:2460–4.

[34] Kim Y, Yoshimura N, Masuda H, et al. Antimuscarinic agents exhibit local inhibitory effects on muscarinic receptors in bladder-afferent pathways. Urology 2005;65:238–42.

[35] Masuda H, Hayashi Y, Masuda N, et al. Roles of bladder muscarinic receptors in the regulation of storage function in rats. J Urol 2005;173:149.

[36] Gillespie JI, Harvey IJ, Drake MJ. Agonist and nerve induced phasic activity in the isolated whole bladder of the guinea pig. Evidence for two types of bladder activity. Exp Physiol 2003;88:343–57.

[37] Gillespie JI. The autonomous bladder: a view of the origin of bladder overactivity and sensory urge. BJU Int 2004;93:478–83.

[38] Wiseman OJ, Brady CM, Hussain IF, et al. The ultrastructure of bladder lamina propria nerves in healthy subjects and patients with detrusor hyperreflexia. J Urol 2002;168:2040–5.

[39] Wiseman OJ, Fowler CJ, Landon DN. The role of the human bladder lamina propria myofibroblast. BJU Int 2003;89:89–93.

[40] Sanders KM. A case for interstitial cells of Cajal as pacemakers and mediators of neurotransmission in the gastrointestinal tract. Gastroenterology 1996;111:492–515.

[41] Sui JP, Rothery S, Dupont E, et al. Gap junctions and connexin expression in human suburothelial interstitial cells. BJU Int 2002;90:118–29.

[42] Salas NA, Smith CP, Kiss S, et al. Intravesical cholinergic receptor activated spinal ATP release in normal and chronic spinal cord injured rats. J Urol 2005;173:45.

[43] Chaiyaprasithi B, Mang CF, Kilbinger H, et al. Inhibition of human detrusor contraction by a urothelium derived factor. J Urol 2003;170:1897–900.

[44] Shimizu I, Kawashima K, Hosoki K. Urodynamics in acetone-induced cystitis of anesthetized rats. Neurourol Urodyn 1999;18:115–27.

[45] Shimizu I, Kawashima K, Ishi D, et al. Effects of AH-9700, (+)-pentazocine, DTG and oxybutynin on micturition in anesthetized rats with acetone-induced cystitis. Life Sci 2001;69:1691–7.

[46] Shenot PJ, Chancellor MB, Rivas DA, et al. In-vivo whole bladder response to anticholinergic and musculotropic agents in spinal cord injured rats. J Spinal Cord Med 1997;20:31–5.

[47] Sasaki Y, Hamada K, Yamazaki C, et al. Effects of NS-21, an anticholinergic drug with calcium antagonistic activity, on lower urinary tract function in a rat model of urinary frequency. Int J Urol 1997;4:401–6.

[48] Angelico P, Valasco C, Guarneri L, et al. Urodynamic effects of oxybutynin and tolterodine in conscious and anesthetized rats under different cystometrographic conditions. BMC Pharmacol 2005;5:1–17.

[49] Zhang X, Igawa Y, Ishizuka O, et al. Effects of resiniferatoxin desensitization of capsaicin-sensitive afferents of detrusor over-activity induced by intravesical capsaicin, acetic acid or ATP in conscious rats. Naunyn Schmiedebergs Arch Pharmacol 2003;367:473–9.

[50] Andersson KE, Chapple CR. Oxybutynin and the overactive bladder. World J Urol 2001;19:319–23.

[51] Kachur JF, Peterson JS, Carter JP, et al. R and S enantiomers of oxybutynin: pharmacological effects in

guinea pig bladder and intestine. J Pharmacol Exp Ther 1988;247:867–72.

[52] Buyse G, Waldeck K, Verpoorten C, et al. Intravesical oxybutynin for neurogenic bladder dysfunction: less systemic side effects due to reduced first pass metabolism. J Urol 1998;160:892–6.

[53] Lose G, Norgaard JP. Intravesical oxybutynin for treating incontinence resulting from an overactive detrusor. BJU Int 2001;87:767–73.

[54] De Wachter S, Wyndaele J-J. Intravesical oxybutynin: a local anesthetic effect on bladder C afferents. J Urol 2003;169:1892–5.

[55] Yokoyama O, Yusup A, Miwa Y, et al. Effects of tolterodine on an overactive bladder depend on suppression of C-fiber bladder afferent activity in rats. J Urol 2005;174:2032–6.

[56] Meglasson MD, Clark MA, Wheeler GJ, et al. Neurokinin-2 (NK-2) receptor antagonism by tolterodine tartrate. J Urol 2003;169:41.

[57] Burgard EC, Bookout AL, McKenna DG, et al. Modulation of calcium currents in bladder sensory neurons by antimuscarinic agents. J Urol 2005; 170:41.

[58] Ozturk H, Onen A, Guneli E, et al. Effects of methoctramine on bladder overactivity in a rat model. Urology 2003;61:671–6.

[59] Yamanishi T, Chapple CR, Yasuda K, et al. The role of M_2 muscarinic receptor subtypes in mediating contraction of the pig bladder base after cyclic adenosine monophosphate elevation and/or selective M_3 inactivation. J Urol 2002;167:397–401.

[60] Kim Y, Yoshimura N, Masuda H, et al. Intravesical instillation of human urine after oral administration of trospium, tolterodine and oxybutynin in a rat model of detrusor overactivity. BJU Int 2005;97:400–3.

[61] Pak RW, Petrou SP, Staskin DR. Trospium chloride: a quaternary amine with unique pharmacological properties. Curr Urol Rep 2003;4:436–40.

ELSEVIER
SAUNDERS

Urol Clin N Am 33 (2006) 519–530

UROLOGIC
CLINICS
of North America

Local Drug Delivery to Bladder Using Technology Innovations

Pradeep Tyagi, PhD[a],*, Shachi Tyagi, MD[a],
Jonathan Kaufman, PhD, MBA[b], Leaf Huang, PhD[c],
Fernando de Miguel, PhD[a]

[a]*Department of Urology, University of Pittsburgh School of Medicine, Kaufmann Medical Building,
Suite 700, 3471 Fifth Avenue, Pittsburgh, PA 15213-3221, USA*
[b]*Lipella Pharmaceuticals, Pittsburgh, PA, USA*
[c]*School of Pharmacy, University of North Carolina at Chapel Hill, Chapel Hill, NC, USA*

Pharmacologic management of diseases typically affecting the bladder frequently require drug administration by way of a catheter into the bladder. Drug delivery by this route, referred to as intravesical delivery, allows drug delivery at the desired site with reduced systemic side effects compared with oral delivery systems [1]. These characteristics ensure maximal therapeutic benefit to occur at the desired site and provide genuine benefits for patients who have morbid adverse effects from oral administration. Bladder cancer, cystitis, and neurogenic bladder are the common conditions managed by this form of drug administration.

Intravesical delivery of bacillus Calmette-Guérin (BCG) is considered first-line treatment for superficial bladder cancer, and in most patients, the complete response rate from BCG is slightly higher for carcinoma in situ than for papillary tumors [2]. The intravesical route is not the predominant route for other ailments of the bladder, but nearly half of overactive bladder patients cannot tolerate oral administration of

anticholinergic agents because of troublesome side effects such as excessive dry mouth, constipation, or blurred vision [3]. The systemic side effects of the most widely used anticholinergic (oxybutynin) are believed to be caused by the high plasma level of its active metabolite, N-desethyl-oxybutynin [4]. Delivery of oxybutynin directly into the bladder in such patients can bring about a local anticholinergic effect, with improved drug tolerability and patient compliance [5].

Most of the newer macromolecular drugs have poor bioavailability when administered orally and often fail to induce a clinical response. Drug delivery by the intravesical route can overcome intrinsic shortcomings of oral therapy such as first-pass metabolism or other drug- or formulation-specific vagaries in absorption, metabolism, and renal excretion. For example, the oral route requires thrice-daily administration for 6 months of the cytoprotective drug misoprostol to achieve therapeutic benefit in interstitial cystitis (IC) patients [6]. Low amounts of drug excreted in the urine following oral administration are probably responsible for the prolonged regimen required for therapeutic benefit. The pharmacokinetics of drugs instilled into the bladder have recently been reviewed [7]. The need for a higher concentration of drug inside the bladder can be solved by instillation, and an improvement in efficacy from local delivery can be made by applying the technologic innovations covered in this article.

This research was funded by grants from the National Institutes of Health (DK 068556), DK 066138, and the Fishbein Family Foundation (CURE-IC).

* Corresponding author. Department of Urology, W326, Montefiore Hospital, 3459 Fifth Avenue, Pittsburgh, PA 15213.

E-mail address: prtst2@pitt.edu (P. Tyagi).

History of intravesical drug delivery

The drastic reduction in the incidence of systemic side effects by the intravesical route has allowed the use of very toxic agents. The first human application of drug delivery using a urethral catheter can be traced back to more than a century when Herring [8] tried instilling silver nitrate for the treatment of superficial bladder cancer. Nearly 60 years later in 1967, dimethyl sulfoxide (DMSO) was instilled for treating refractory cases of IC [9,10]. DMSO was approved by the US Food and Drug Administration in 1978 as a 50% solution with primary indication for treating IC [11]. Another member from the list of toxic agents instilled into the bladder is BCG, indicated in the treatment of refractory bladder cancer [12]. Treatment with BCG delays tumor progression and significantly decreases the need for subsequent cystectomy, with improved overall survival rates [13]. BCG triggers a variety of local immune responses including induction of proliferator-activated receptor γ (PPARγ) that appear to correlate with antitumor activity [14]. A member of the nuclear receptor superfamily of ligand-activated transcription factors, PPARγ is expressed in normal urothelium and is known to be involved in cell growth, differentiation, and inflammatory processes [15]. The immunomodulatory activity of BCG also prompted its evaluation for immunotherapy of IC, and BCG produced a favorable outcome in refractory IC patients [16,17]. The ability of prostaglandins to cause smooth muscle contraction was exploited for treating detrusor underactivity or underactive bladder using intravesical therapy of prostaglandin E_2 [18].

Barriers to urothelium and intravesical therapy

Drugs instilled into the bladder have to cross a watertight barrier between blood and urine formed by the bladder lining to elicit any effect. The cell layer lining the interior of the bladder is called urothelium or transistional cell epithelium and forms a barrier that is equally effective in blocking the entry of urine contents and instilled drugs [19,20]. Examination of umbrella cells lying at the luminal surface of urothelium using electron microscopy showed that hexagonally packed uroplakins cover most of the apical side of umbrella cells [21]. The six subunits of each particle are joined together to form a complete hexagonal ring, with lipids contained in its central cavity. The low permeability–barrier urothelium is believed to crop up from the peculiar protein array

and the tight junctions between umbrella cells [22,23]. The absorption of drug is further restricted by the glycosaminoglycan (GAG) layer on the surface of umbrella cells [24].

In hypothetical terms, the barrier of urothelium may prove to be tougher than the blood-brain barrier because the former is made up of generally stronger epithelial cells and the latter by generally weaker endothelial cells. Weekly drug instillation into the bladder demonstrated that drug concentration in bladder tissue is linearly dependent on the concentration of drug in urine. The linear relationship suggests that passive diffusion is the only mode of membrane transport available for the intravesical route of drug administration [25]. Because concentration gradient is the sole driving force available for drug absorption, it is logical to expect an increase in drug transport with improvement in the concentration gradient. Complete bladder emptying just before dose administration and restricted fluid intake can be used to mitigate the influence of the kidney on intravesical therapy [26]. This method reduces the immediate dilution of drug concentration by residual urine in the bladder and diminishes the steady dilution by constant urine production during the time period for which instillation is still in the bladder. Increased concentration in urine can improve the efficacy of a drug acting in the bladder without significant enhancement in toxicity [26]. Using such techniques, enhanced penetration of mitomycin C across bladder urothelium in a recent phase III trial nearly doubled the recurrence-free rate in patients who had superficial bladder cancer [27].

Intravesical treatment of interstitial cystitis

Little is known about the pathogenesis of IC, which leaves most treatments including intravesical treatments of IC to be symptomatic. The most consistent finding in IC patients, however, involves dysfunction of the superficial layer of extracellular matrix (GAG layer) and localization of a high number of activated mast cells in the bladder [28,29]. A superficial layer of GAG is covalently attached to the membrane proteins of umbrella cells residing in the topmost layer of urothelium cells of the bladder [22]. Hyaluronic acid is an important component in the urothelium, and sodium hyaluronate has been instilled in IC patients for possible replenishment of bladder GAG in the treatment of IC [30]. Hyaluronic acid inhibits leukocyte migration, aggregation, and adherence of immune complexes to polymorphonuclear cells. Another GAG analog effective in approximately 50% of IC patients following its instillation is heparin [31]. A recent study showed that intravesically administered fluorescent-labeled chondroitin sulfate in mouse bladder coated the damaged bladder surface, explaining its clinical efficacy [32].

Intravesical treatment of particularly severe chronic IC requires addressing the significant upregulation of afferents in the bladder [33]. C-fiber afferents are considered to be responsible for the aberrant micturition reflex in IC. These C-fiber afferents are believed to be silent under normal conditions but are activated after bladder irritation and spinal cord injury [34]. A viable treatment approach that is gaining ground is the downregulation of sensory nerves by treating them with neurotoxin such as capsaicin or resiniferatoxin [33]. Administration of vanilloids by the intravesical route restricts the potent action of vanilloids to the afferent fibers in the bladder wall, thereby avoiding possible systemic neurotoxicity [35]. The hydrophobic nature of these neurotoxins, however, necessitates the use of ethanol as a cosolvent and saline as the vehicle for instillation into the bladder. Ethanol is well known to induce inflammation in different tissues [36]. Recent studies have demonstrated the superiority of nonalcoholic solvents for vanilloids over alcohol solvents [37,38]. Liposomes have also been used to try to overcome the aqueous insolubility of vanilloids.

Instillation of liposomes

The approach of intravesical drug delivery is amenable to the modulation of release and absorption characteristics of the instilled drugs through its coupling to carrier particles such as microspheres, nanoparticles, liposomes, and so forth. Liposomes were first studied in England in 1961 by Bangham [39] and have since become a versatile tool of study in biology, biochemistry, and medicine. Liposomes are artificial spherical vesicles consisting of an aqueous core enclosed in one or more phospholipid layers. They have been used as intravesical drug carriers after being loaded with a great variety of molecules such as small drug molecules, proteins, nucleotides, and even plasmids [40–43]. The flexibility of their compositions makes liposomes a versatile drug delivery vehicle. The use of multilamellar liposomes proved favorable in cell culture studies, and the antiproliferative capacity of interferon-α in a resistant bladder cancer cell line was improved by using liposomes as a delivery vehicle [44]. Instillation of liposome-encapsulated radiolabeled interferon-α or radiolabeled liposomes into mouse bladder was able to achieve localized therapy with negligible penetration to other organs [45]. Previously, liposomes have proven to improve the aqueous solubility of hydrophobic drugs such as taxol and amphotericin [46]. A recent study reported from the authors' laboratory used liposomes as a vehicle for capsaicin and evaluated their potential as a vehicle for intravesical delivery in rats [38]. Efficacy of a new delivery system for capsaicin was evaluated by measuring micturition reflex in normal rats under urethane anesthesia (Fig. 1).

Awake micturition in such rats with an intact neuraxis is dependent on a spinobulbospinal reflex activated by A delta–fiber bladder afferents, and facilitatory action of capsaicin-sensitive nerves on micturition threshold is more evident in anesthetized rats than awake rats because capsaicin-resistant bladder afferents are more sensitive to the depressant action of urethane than the capsaicin-sensitive afferents [47]. The cystometrogram (CMG) tracings shown in Fig. 2 illustrate that liposomes were able to deliver capsaicin with efficacy similar to ethanolic saline. Tissue histology and morphology studies, however, revealed that toxicity to the bladder was drastically reduced [38]. As reported previously, liposomes can form a film on cell surfaces and have been tested as possible therapeutic agents to promote wound healing [48]. Such reports prompted the evaluation of liposomes devoid of any drug in a rat model of bladder hyperactivity. Liposomes alone were able to partially reverse the high bladder frequency induced by protamine sulfate/potassium chloride (Fig. 3) [49]. These observations suggest that liposomes might enhance the barrier properties of a dysfunctional urothelium and increase resistance to irritant penetration. Liposomes are prepared from the phospholipids that are the major component of cell membranes. Presumably, instillation of liposomes adds to the permeability barrier of urothelium by their adherence to the injured surface (Fig. 4).

Overcoming barriers to intravescial therapy

Inadequate intravesical drug delivery often happens due to the poor penetration of drug through the urothelium. In addition to concentration gradient, factors that can influence transvesical (across urothelium) transport are the molecular weight of the drug and the pH of

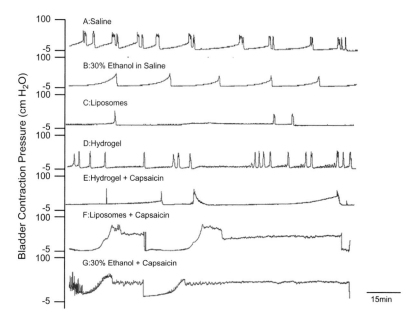

Fig. 1. Representative tracings of CMG after instillation of normal saline showing periodic micturition events under urethane anesthesia. Tracing B and tracing C represent 30% ethanol-treated rats and liposome-treated rats, respectively, in absence of capsaicin, revealing the dissimilar effects of ethanol and liposomes on bladder afferents by decrease in bladder contraction frequency. Tracing D and tracing E are hydrogel-treated rats in the absence of and in the presence of capsaicin, respectively, revealing a decrease in bladder contraction frequency in the presence of capsaicin. Tracing F and tracing G are from rats treated with liposomes and 30% ethanol, respectively, in presence of capsaicin, showing complete blockade of micturition reflex in both cases. A raised plateau of bladder contraction pressure reflects urinary retention.

the instilled solution [50]. Unsuccessful drug delivery using conventional formulations and a resistant drug target are the two main reasons attributed for the undesirable outcomes from intravesical drug delivery. Therapy by the intravesical route can be improved by helping drugs to cross the permeability barrier of urothelium by physical alteration (iontophoresis and electroporation) and by chemical alteration (DMSO, saponin).

Physical approaches

There is a plethora of reports on enhancing transdermal drug transport with the use of electromotive drug administration (EMDA) or iontophoresis [51,52]. In animal studies, very low voltages of electric current have been used for EMDA, which is a technique that drives drugs (mitomycin C, oxybutynin, and bethanechol) and dyes deep into the muscular layers of the

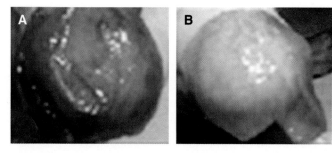

Fig. 2. Bladder morphology pictures after instillation of capsaicin in saline with 30% ethanol (*A*) and in liposomes (*B*). Redness in panel *A* indicates inflammation. Note the absence of redness in panel *B*.

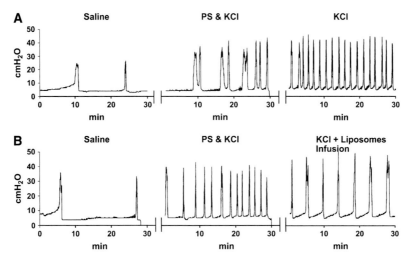

Fig. 3. Effect of liposomes in a bladder injury model induced by protamine sulfate (PS) and irritated by potassium chloride (KCl). (*A*) Liposomes were coadministered with KCl as shown by the CMG tracing in the bottom panel to reduce the bladder contraction frequency. (*B*) Bottom panel shows the CMG of the untreated rat bladder, indicating bladder hyperactivity.

bladder wall. Anesthesia suitable for transurethral resection of bladder tumors, bladder neck incision, and hydrodistension of the bladder has been accomplished clinically after EMDA of local anesthetics by applying an electric current in the range of 20 mA for a few minutes [53,54]. A recent clinical trial combined BCG treatment with increased bladder uptake of mitomycin C through EMDA to improve the response rate in 212 patients who had stage pT1 bladder cancer [55]. In addition to EMDA, the permeability of mitomycin across urothelium was increased by BCG-induced inflammation in the bladder [55]. In most patients, EMDA causes only minor local irritation with no systemic side effects, but a recent case report of transient ischemic attack was reported from Germany following EMDA in elderly men suffering from cystitis [56]. The investigators suspected epinephrine to be cause of ischemic attack after intravesical EMDA. Electroporation is another approach that uses an electrical field to increase tissue permeability. It differs from iontophoresis in that it uses comparatively higher voltage for improving intravesical delivery of drugs in the treatment of bladder carcinoma [57]. In a recent study, the efficacy of intravesically administered mitomycin C on small superficial tumors was enhanced by using local microwave-induced hyperthermia [58].

Chemical approaches

It has been reported that absorption of chemotherapeutic drugs including paclitaxel and pirarubicin can be enhanced by DMSO instillation [59,60]. Sasaki and colleagues [61] reported that intravesical instillation of saponin before administration of the anticancer drug 4'-O-tetrahydropyranyldoxorubicin (THP) can cause

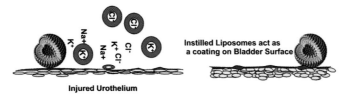

Fig. 4. Illustration of the underlying protective effects of liposomes on the bladder surface injured by protamine and irritated by potassium chloride (*left*). Instilled liposomes form a protective coating on the injured bladder surface (*right*).

vacuolization and swelling of superficial cells. The concentration of THP in bladder tissue was significantly higher than that of untreated animals, but in plasma, no difference was revealed [61,62].

Currently, treatment of severe overactive bladder requires cystoscopic-guided injections of botulinum toxin type A at 20 to 30 different sites of detrusor in the bladder. Botulinum toxin type A provides its long-lasting effect by blocking the release of acetylcholine from nerve endings to impair involuntary detrusor contractions [63]. Instillation of this high molecular weight protein toxin requires improvement in permeability for its absorption. The absorption of this dangerous toxin has to be localized because any systemic absorption can prove fatal; this must be taken into consideration in the development of any future delivery techniques. Pretreatment of urothelium with protamine sulfate to improve the permeability for botulinum toxin type A has been attempted in rats [64,65]. The cationic nature of protamine sulfate allows a charge interaction with the anionically charged GAG layer, leading to a slight increase in permeability of the urothelium [66].

Recently, certain peptides called "cell penetrating peptides" or "protein transduction domains" have been shown to possess the ability to translocate large macromolecular drugs across the blood-brain barrier and membranes of other cells [67]. These peptides, however, lack the ability to be cell selective and are therefore a poor choice for systemic drug targeting [68]. The authors examined the effect of using the short-length TransActivator of Transcription (TAT) peptide derived from HIV for intravesical administration of large macromolecular drugs such as peptide nucleic acid (PNA). Antisense agents that inhibit genes at the mRNA level are attractive tools for genomewide studies and drug target validation, and PNAs have been used for their antisense effect in various studies because they form stable duplexes with the target mRNA and arrest translation of proteins [69]. PNA has superior binding properties and higher stability in biologic media such as urine over a wide pH range compared with traditional oligonucleotides and ribozymes [70]. The eleven–amino acid TAT peptide was coupled to 18mer antisense PNA by Fmoc chemistry, and similar chemistry was used to tag a fluorescent rhodamine probe. Translocation across rat urothelium was visualized by confocal microscopy of the red fluorescence of rhodamine in bladder sections [71].

Sustained drug delivery

Conventional formulations are maintained in the bladder for only short periods—typically less than 2 hours—and often, patients do not completely respond or the response is highly variable among patients. The drug exposure at the urothelium rarely lasts beyond the first voiding of urine after instillation of conventional formulations. Sustained intravesical delivery of drugs can ensure continuous presence of drug in the bladder without the need for intermittent catheterization, and drug concentration in the bladder can be constant without any peaks and valleys. It is also plausible to expect an increase in efficacy with the increased duration of direct contact between the drug and the abnormal urothelium [45]. Attempts to overcome this inherent drawback of intravesical instillation have been reported from various laboratories.

A simple and sensible approach for sustained intravesical delivery is prolonged infusion into the bladder. This technique has often been applied for achieving slow and sustained release of drugs inside the bladder. Prolonged instillation of resiniferatoxin was recently demonstrated as a feasible procedure for treating neurogenic bladder [72]. Resiniferatoxin was infused through a sovrapubic 5F monopigtail catheter for 10 days at the flow rate of 25 μL/h with the help of an infusion pump. Patients were evaluated 30 days after the end of the infusion and after 3 months. A 30% decrease in frequency and a threefold reduction of nocturia with significant reduction of symptoms of pelvic pain for at least 6 months after the end of the infusion were observed. Similar approaches have previously been applied for local therapy of prostaglandins in the treatment of cyclophosphamide-induced cystitis in patients [73]. Cystitis is a major complication from the high-dose cyclophosphamide regimen used against allogeneic or autologous bone marrow transplantation. A 100-mL irrigation of 5 μg/mL of prostaglandin E_2 into the bladder for 3 hours completely freed a 4-year-old patient from all symptoms within 24 hours [74]. Intravescial infusion of carboprost had a success rate of over 60% in patients who had hemorrhagic cystitis after marrow transplantation [75]. Response was achieved by infusing carboprost at 2 μg/mL for an hour four times a day with a fivefold dose escalation every 24 hours.

Forming a drug depot inside the bladder appears to be an attractive option versus prolonged infusion. Aqueous solutions of poly (ethylene glycol-b-[DL-lactic acid-co-glycolic acid]-

b-ethylene glycol) (PEG-PLGA-PEG) triblock copolymers form a free-flowing solution at room temperature and become a viscous gel at body temperature (37°C) [76]. Its formulation does not require organic solvents, and products from its bioerosion of the biocompatible polymer are nontoxic polyethylene glycol, glycolic acid, and lactic acid [77]. Such a thermosensitive hydrogel formed by PEG-PLGA-PEG has been used for in situ gel formation for a depot of hydrophobic and hydrophilic drugs following subcutaneous administration in rats [78]. The triblock copolymer was used for sustaining the residence time of hydrophobic drugs in rat bladder after its instillation at room temperature. The kinetics of drug excretion was studied by fluorescence measurement of urine after instilling fluorescein isothiocyanate–loaded hydrogel. The increased urine concentration over a period of time implies increased penetration into the bladder tissue [25]. The therapeutic benefit of sustained delivery afforded by the thermosensitive hydrogel was demonstrated by delivering misoprostol, an anti-inflammatory drug. It was able to protect the bladder against cyclophosphamide-induced cystitis [79].

Bioadhesion

The presence of a mucin–glycocalyx domain in urotheliun can be used for prolonging the residence time of drugs by exploiting the approach of bioadhesion [80]. Bioadhesion or mucoadhesion defines the interaction between a biologic surface such as bladder mucosa (urothelium) and the polymer. The term *mucoadhesion* is used specifically when adhesion involves mucous coating and an adhesive polymeric device, whereas epithelial cell–specific bioadhesion is termed *cytoadhesion*. Adhesion with mucin and mucoadhesive polymers is usually based on molecular attractive and repulsive forces; in contrast, adhesion to cell surfaces involves highly specific receptor-mediated interactions.

The process is said to occur through the following steps:

1. Initial physical interaction or mutual wetting between the polymer and the surface.
2. Interpenetration of the polymer and the components of the GAG layer on the urothelium.
3. Electrostatic interactions, hydrogen-bond formation, and van der Waals forces between the polymer and biologic surface.

Mucoadhesive materials are generally hydrophilic polymers that swell significantly in contact with water and eventually undergo complete dissolution. Also called wet adhesives, these hydrophilic polymers adhere to the mucosal surface after wetting and can be categorized into the following classes: anionic polymers such as sodium carboxymethyl cellulose and sodium alginate, cationic polymers such as chitosan and dextrans, nonionic polymers such as polyvinylpyrollidone, and cellulose derivatives such as hydroxypropylmethyl cellulose. The bioadhesive strength of a polymer increases with its molecular weight because the extent of interpenetration and molecular entanglement seems to be determined by the length of the polymer chain. Polyethylene glycol can be used as an adhesion promoter between polymer and GAG by diffusion of the polyethylene glycol chains into the polymeric networks of GAG and the polymer [81].

The coupling of bioadhesion characteristics to the carrier particles such as microspheres can lend additional advantages to these delivery systems, such as efficient absorption and enhanced bioavailability of the drugs due to increased surface area for a given volume of drug and a much more intimate contact with the mucus layer. For example, chitosan microspheres were able to increase the ocular residence time and decrease the frequent administration of acyclovir by way of ophthalmic route [82]. Similar expectations have motivated the use of bioadhesives for improving intravesical drug delivery [83]. The application of bioadhesives in intravesical drug delivery should be able to fulfill three main criteria: readily adhere after instillation to the urothelium; be unobtrusive to the micturition function; and be retained in place for at least several hours. Chitosan and polycarbophil retain good adhesion after full hydration, and their ability to increase adhesion of a hydrophilic drug to urothelium was evaluated using isolated porcine urinary bladder [84]. Drug distribution in to the bladder wall was determined by sectioning the frozen bladder and extracting the drug from tissue slices for analysis [84].

The first generation of mucoadhesive polymers lacked specificity, such as the suspensions of algin salts that simply swelled and formed an adherent viscous layer on contact with the mucosa. In contrast to classic mucoadhesion, which relies on nonspecific interpenetration of polymer chains and mucus, the anchoring of plant lectins, bacterial adhesions, and antibodies on the surface of the microspheres can increase the therapeutic benefit. Any ligand with a high binding affinity for mucin can be covalently linked to the microspheres and expected to influence the binding of microspheres to the mucus surface. The lectin–sugar interaction may represent a step forward toward drug delivery across mucosal surfaces. Lectins are proteins of nonimmune origin that bind to carbohydrates specifically and noncovalently [85]. The epithelial lining of most visceral organs is covered with a mucous layer, and lectins attached to a drug delivery system can interact with the highly glycosylated proteins making up the mucin molecules of the mucus. In addition to lectin-mediated drug delivery systems, the carbohydrate specificity of mucus is used by microorganisms to adhere to the gut or to bladder mucosa. Bacteria use lectin–sugar interactions to adhere to the sterile surface of the bladder and cause urinary tract infection, but in the gut, the same bacterial species constitutes the normal microflora.

Postoperative chemotherapy in mice was successful with bioadhesive carriers based on polymers such as algin, chitosan, and fibrinogen [86]. Mitomycin C–loaded alginate and chitosan bioadhsive carriers were evaluated in the murine bladder cancer model [86]. Intravesical administration of poly (methylidene malonate-2.1.2) bioadhesive microspheres achieved controlled release of the paclitaxel at the urothelium/urine interface of mouse bladder [83]. Spherical 5-μm thick microspheres adhered to the mouse urothelium for up to 2 days and mice that had bladder cancer survived for a significantly longer time following instillation of bioadhesive microspheres loaded with 5% w/w paclitaxel compared with similar doses of the conventional paclitaxel formulation.

Daily micturition events (12–15 events) could not flush out the microspheres from mouse bladder [87]. In another study employing a similar approach, a fibrinogen-based bioadhesive loaded with 5-fluorouracil was used for preventing tumor recurrence in the resected tumor beds of mouse bladder [88]. Storage-Phosphor autoradiography was used to quantify drug retention in the bladder after administration, which showed more than a twofold increase for the bioadhesive drug over drug solution alone.

Temporal and spatial monitoring of instilled microparticles is possible with MRI [89]. Polymeric microparticles were encapsulated with MRI contrast agent gadolinium diethylenetriamine pentaacetic acid for measuring T1 relaxation rate of particles until 5 days after instillation. Retention of doxorubin in dog bladder was increased by instilling microparticles called magnetic targeted carriers and composed of metallic iron and doxorubicin adsorbed onto activated carbon. An externally applied magnetic field was used to achieve extended retention of magnetic targeted carriers following instillation [90]. Another gelatin-based delivery system released drugs for 12 days in the rabbit bladder [91].

Intravesical delivery of oxybutynin has proved suitable for patients who have overactive bladder suffering from side effects of the metabolite N-desethyl-oxybutynin following oral administration [5]. The local delivery of oxybutynin into bladder by employing the approach of mucoadhesion achieved partial clinical success in a case study involving six patients [4,92]. The mucoadhesive solution of oxybutynin was prepared by adding hydroxypropylcellulose to the oxybutynin chloride solution (5% w/w) that was instilled twice daily at a dose of 0.5 mg/mL using the catheter used for bladder emptying [92]. CMG was performed on patients before starting the treatment and at 1 week and 3 years after the first instillation of oxybutynin. A significant increase in bladder capacity was observed in four of the six patients. This intravesical oxybutynin therapy is thought to depend on three mechanisms that prevent or improve urge incontinence: the direct effect on bladder muscle, the topical anesthetic effect, and the indirect effect of absorbed oxybutynin and its metabolites [4].

Future perspectives

Recent years have seen an increased interest in nanotechnology, a new technique that involves the creation and manipulation of materials at nanoscale levels to create products that exhibit novel properties. For example, rapid-release, paclitaxel-loaded, gelatin nanoparticles with a particle size ranging from 600 to 1000 nm were recently designed for intravesical bladder cancer therapy [93]. The paclitaxel nanoparticles showed significant activity against human bladder cancer cells and resulted in higher tissue concentrations compared with existing vehicles. Drug exposure in the bladder can be successfully increased using the approach of bioadesion. Before bioadhesion caught the fancy of drug-delivery scientists, this powerful approach had been exploited by *Escherichia coli* for adhesion to the bladder mucosa. Urinary tract infections are initiated by adhesion of uropathogenic *E coli* to uroplakin receptors in the uroepithelium by way of the FimH adhesin located at the tips of type 1 pili. Perhaps we can learn from *E coli* and design a drug-delivery system that uses bacterial adhesion factors to increase adhesion to epithelial surfaces.

Summary

Intravesical drug delivery is a highly promising alternative when disease has become refractory to treatment with drugs administered from other routes. The recent advances covered in this article have been successful in overcoming the drawbacks of this route in preclinical studies (Fig. 5). The therapeutic benefit from newer therapeutic entities such as botulinum toxin, cannabinoids, and vanilloids against overactive bladder and IC can be augmented by using newer delivery systems. The new approach of liposomes holds tremendous promise as a therapy and a drug delivery platform for drugs administered intravesically. The authors look forward to the day when liposomes can be tested in clinical trials to help patients who have painful bladder syndrome and to improve bladder drug delivery.

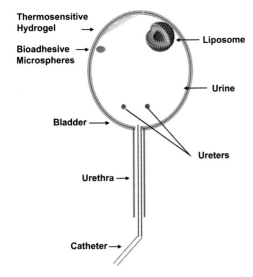

Fig. 5. Illustration of the newer drug-delivery system instilled into the bladder, based on innovative technology. Liposomes and microspheres with bioadhesive coating allow them to adhere to the bladder surface. The thermosensitive hydrogel forms a viscous semisolid gel inside the bladder after being instilled as a fluid.

References

[1] Dmochowski RR, Staskin DR. Advances in drug delivery: improved bioavailability and drug effect. Curr Urol Rep 2002;3(6):439–44.

[2] de Reijke TM, Kurth KH, Sylvester RJ, et al. Bacillus Calmette-Guerin versus epirubicin for primary, secondary or concurrent carcinoma in situ of the bladder: results of a European Organization for the Research and Treatment of Cancer–Genito-Urinary Group Phase III Trial (30906). J Urol 2005;173(2):405–9.

[3] Wein AJ. Practical uropharmacology. Urol Clin North Am 1991;18(2):269–81.

[4] Abramov Y, Sand PK. Oxybutynin for treatment of urge urinary incontinence and overactive bladder: an updated review. Expert Opin Pharmacother 2004; 5(11):2351–9.

[5] Buyse G, Waldeck K, Verpoorten C, et al. Intravesical oxybutynin for neurogenic bladder dysfunction: less systemic side effects due to reduced first pass metabolism. J Urol 1998;160(3 Pt 1):892–6.

[6] Kelly JD, Young MR, Johnston SR, et al. Clinical response to an oral prostaglandin analogue in patients with interstitial cystitis. Eur Urol 1998;34(1): 53–6.

[7] Highley MS, van Oosterom AT, Maes RA, et al. Intravesical drug delivery. Pharmacokinetic and clinical considerations. Clin Pharmacokinet 1999; 37(1):59–73.

[8] Herring H. The treatment of vesical papilloma by injections. BMJ 1903;2:1398.

[9] Stewart BH, Persky L, Kiser WS. The use of dimethyl sulfoxide (DMSO) in the treatment of interstitial cystitis. J Urol 1967;98(6):671–2.

[10] Parkin J, Shea C, Sant GR. Intravesical dimethyl sulfoxide (DMSO) for interstitial cystitis—a practical approach. Urology 1997;49(5A Suppl):105–7.

[11] Shirley SW, Stewart BH, Mirelman S. Dimethyl sulfoxide in treatment of inflammatory genitourinary disorders. Urology 1978;11(3):215–20.

[12] Joudi FN, O'Donnell MA. Second-line intravesical therapy versus cystectomy for bacille Calmette-Guerin (BCG) failures. Curr Opin Urol 2004;14(5): 271–5.

[13] Kassouf W, Kamat AM. Current state of immunotherapy for bladder cancer. Expert Rev Anticancer Ther 2004;4(6):1037–46.

[14] Lodillinsky C, Umerez MS, Jasnis MA, et al. Bacillus Calmette-Guerin induces the expression of peroxisome proliferator-activated receptor gamma in bladder cancer cells. Int J Mol Med 2006;17(2): 269–73.

[15] Guan Y. Targeting peroxisome proliferator-activated receptors (PPARs) in kidney and urologic disease. Minerva Urol Nefrol 2002;54(2):65–79.

[16] Zeidman EJ, Helfrick B, Pollard C, et al. Bacillus Calmette-Guerin immunotherapy for refractory interstitial cystitis. Urology 1994;43(1):121–4.

[17] Lukban JC, Whitmore KE, Sant GR. Current management of interstitial cystitis. Urol Clin North Am 2002;29(3):649–60.

[18] Hindley RG, Brierly RD, Thomas PJ. Prostaglandin E2 and bethanechol in combination for treating detrusor underactivity. BJU Int 2004;93(1):89–92.

[19] Melicow MM. The urothelium: a battleground for oncogenesis. J Urol 1978;120(1):43–7.

[20] Apodaca G. The uroepithelium: not just a passive barrier. Traffic 2004;5(3):117–28.

[21] Min G, Zhou G, Schapira M, et al. Structural basis of urothelial permeability barrier function as revealed by Cryo-EM studies of the 16 nm uroplakin particle. J Cell Sci 2003;116(Pt 20):4087–94.

[22] Hurst RE, Zebrowski R. Identification of proteoglycans present at high density on bovine and human bladder luminal surface. J Urol 1994;152(5 Pt 1):1641–5.

[23] Born M, Pahner I, Ahnert-Hilger G, et al. The maintenance of the permeability barrier of bladder facet cells requires a continuous fusion of discoid vesicles with the apical plasma membrane. Eur J Cell Biol 2003;82(7):343–50.

[24] Parsons CL, Mulholland SG, Anwar H. Antibacterial activity of bladder surface mucin duplicated by exogenous glycosaminoglycan (heparin). Infect Immun 1979;24(2):552–7.

[25] Gao X, Au JL, Badalament RA, et al. Bladder tissue uptake of mitomycin C during intravesical therapy is linear with drug concentration in urine. Clin Cancer Res 1998;4(1):139–43.

[26] Au JL, Badalament RA, Wientjes MG, et al. Methods to improve efficacy of intravesical mitomycin C: results of a randomized phase III trial. J Natl Cancer Inst 2001;93(8):597–604.

[27] Au JL, Jang SH, Wientjes MG. Clinical aspects of drug delivery to tumors. J Control Release 2002;78(1–3):81–95.

[28] Parsons CL, Greene RA, Chung M, et al. Abnormal urinary potassium metabolism in patients with interstitial cystitis. J Urol 2005;173(4):1182–5.

[29] Theoharides TC, Sant GR. A pilot open label study of Cystoprotek(R) in interstitial cystitis. Int J Immunopathol Pharmacol 2005;18(1):183–8.

[30] Daha LK, Riedl CR, Lazar D, et al. Do cystometric findings predict the results of intravesical hyaluronic acid in women with interstitial cystitis? Eur Urol 2005;47(3):393–7.

[31] Parsons CL. Current strategies for managing interstitial cystitis. Expert Opin Pharmacother 2004;5(2):287–93.

[32] Kyker KD, Coffman J, Hurst RE. Exogenous glycosaminoglycans coat damaged bladder surfaces in experimentally damaged mouse bladder. BMC Urol 2005;5(1):4.

[33] Chancellor MB, Yoshimura N. Treatment of interstitial cystitis. Urology 2004;63(3 Suppl 1):85–92.

[34] Cruz F. Mechanisms involved in new therapies for overactive bladder. Urology 2004;63(3 Suppl 1):65–73.

[35] Ritter S, Dinh TT. Age-related changes in capsaicin-induced degeneration in rat brain. J Comp Neurol 1992;318(1):103–16.

[36] Trevisani M, Gazzieri D, Benvenuti F, et al. Ethanol causes inflammation in the airways by a neurogenic and TRPV1-dependent mechanism. J Pharmacol Exp Ther 2004;309(3):1167–73.

[37] de Seze M, Wiart L, de Seze MP, et al. Intravesical capsaicin versus resiniferatoxin for the treatment of detrusor hyperreflexia in spinal cord injured patients: a double-blind, randomized, controlled study. J Urol 2004;171(1):251–5.

[38] Tyagi P, Chancellor MB, Li Z, et al. Urodynamic and immunohistochemical evaluation of intravesical capsaicin delivery using thermosensitive hydrogel and liposomes. J Urol 2004;171(1):483–9.

[39] Bangham AD. A correlation between surface charge and coagulant action of phospholipids. Nature 1961;192:1197–8.

[40] Tsuruta T, Muraishi O, Katsuyama Y, et al. Liposome encapsulated doxorubicin transfer to the pelvic lymph nodes by endoscopic administration into the bladder wall: a preliminary report. J Urol 1997;157(5):1652–4.

[41] Hikosaka S, Hara I, Miyake H, et al. Antitumor effect of simultaneous transfer of interleukin-12 and interleukin-18 genes and its mechanism in a mouse bladder cancer model. Int J Urol 2004;11(8):647–52.

[42] Nogawa M, Yuasa T, Kimura S, et al. Intravesical administration of small interfering RNA targeting PLK-1 successfully prevents the growth of bladder cancer. J Clin Invest 2005;115(4):978–85.

[43] Zang Z, Mahendran R, Wu Q, et al. Non-viral tumor necrosis factor-alpha gene transfer decreases the incidence of orthotopic bladder tumors. Int J Mol Med 2004;14(4):713–7.

[44] Killion JJ, Fan D, Bucana CD, et al. Augmentation of antiproliferative activity of interferon alfa against human bladder tumor cell lines by encapsulation of interferon alfa within liposomes. J Natl Cancer Inst 1989;81(18):1387–92.

[45] Frangos DN, Killion JJ, Fan D, et al. The development of liposomes containing interferon alpha for the intravesical therapy of human superficial bladder cancer. J Urol 1990;143(6):1252–6.

[46] Ng AW, Wasan KM, Lopez-Berestein G. Liposomal polyene antibiotics. Methods Enzymol 2005;391:304–13.

[47] Maggi CA, Conte B. Effect of urethane anesthesia on the micturition reflex in capsaicin-treated rats. J Auton Nerv Syst 1990;30(3):247–51.

[48] Reimer K, Fleischer W, Brogmann B, et al. Povidone-iodine liposomes—an overview. Dermatology 1997;195(Suppl 2):93–9.

[49] Fraser MO, Chuang YC, Tyagi P, et al. Intravesical liposome administration—a novel treatment for hyperactive bladder in the rat. Urology 2003;61(3): 656–63.

[50] Tammela T, Wein AJ, Monson FC, et al. Urothelial permeability of the isolated whole bladder. Neurourol Urodyn 1993;12(1):39–47.

[51] Schuetz YB, Naik A, Guy RH, et al. Emerging strategies for the transdermal delivery of peptide and protein drugs. Expert Opin Drug Deliv 2005; 2(3):533–48.

[52] Dyson C. Influence of iontophoresis on the permeability of the excised cornea. Arch Ophthal 1949; 42(4):416–21.

[53] Jewett MA, Valiquette L, Sampson HA, et al. Electromotive drug administration of lidocaine as an alternative anesthesia for transurethral surgery. J Urol 1999;161(2):482–5.

[54] Fontanella UA, Rossi CA, Stephen RL. Bladder and urethral anaesthesia with electromotive drug administration (EMDA): a technique for invasive endoscopic procedures. Br J Urol 1997;79(3): 414–20.

[55] Di Stasi SM, Giannantoni A, Giurioli A, et al. Sequential BCG and electromotive mitomycin versus BCG alone for high-risk superficial bladder cancer: a randomised controlled trial. Lancet Oncol 2006; 7(1):43–51.

[56] Hinkel A, Pannek J. Transient ischemic attack after electromotive drug administration for chronic noninfectious cystitis: report of two similar cases. Neurourol Urodyn 2004;23(2):180–2.

[57] Lee CF, Chang SY, Hsieh DS, et al. Treatment of bladder carcinomas using recombinant BCG DNA vaccines and electroporative gene immunotherapy. Cancer Gene Ther 2004;11(3):194–207.

[58] Colombo R, Brausi M, Da Pozzo L, et al. Thermochemotherapy and electromotive drug administration of mitomycin C in superficial bladder cancer eradication. a pilot study on marker lesion. Eur Urol 2001;39(1):95–100.

[59] Chen D, Song D, Wientjes MG, et al. Effect of dimethyl sulfoxide on bladder tissue penetration of intravesical paclitaxel. Clin Cancer Res 2003;9(1): 363–9.

[60] Hashimoto H, Tokunaka S, Sasaki M, et al. Dimethylsulfoxide enhances the absorption of chemotherapeutic drug instilled into the bladder. Urol Res 1992;20(3):233–6.

[61] Sasaki M, Hashimoto H, Yachiku S. [Studies on enhancement of drug absorption through the bladder mucosa]. Nippon Hinyokika Gakkai Zasshi 1994; 85(9):1353–62.

[62] Hashimoto H, Yachiku S, Watabe Y, et al. [Postoperative intravesical installation of tetrahydropyranyladriamycin (THP) and cytosine arabinoside (CA) for superficial bladder cancer: clinical results of prophylactic effects on recurrence]. Gan To Kagaku Ryoho 1994;21(6):833–8.

[63] Chancellor MB. Urgency, botulinum toxin and how botulinum toxin can help urgency. J Urol 2005; 174(3):818.

[64] Vemulakonda VM, Somogyi GT, Kiss S, et al. Inhibitory effect of intravesically applied botulinum toxin A in chronic bladder inflammation. J Urol 2005;173(2):621–4.

[65] Khera M, Somogyi GT, Salas NA, et al. In vivo effects of botulinum toxin A on visceral sensory function in chronic spinal cord-injured rats. Urology 2005;66(1):208–12.

[66] Tzan CJ, Berg JR, Lewis SA. Mammalian urinary bladder permeability is altered by cationic proteins: modulation by divalent cations. Am J Physiol 1994; 267(4 Pt 1):C1013–26.

[67] Schwarze SR, Ho A, Vocero-Akbani A, et al. In vivo protein transduction: delivery of a biologically active protein into the mouse. Science 1999;285(5433): 1569–72.

[68] Astriab-Fisher A, Sergueev D, Fisher M, et al. Conjugates of antisense oligonucleotides with the TAT and antennapedia cell-penetrating peptides: effects on cellular uptake, binding to target sequences, and biologic actions. Pharm Res 2002;19(6):744–54.

[69] Nielsen PE. Gene targeting using peptide nucleic acid. Methods Mol Biol 2005;288:343–58.

[70] Pooga M, Land T, Bartfai T, et al. PNA oligomers as tools for specific modulation of gene expression. Biomol Eng 2001;17(6):183–92.

[71] Tyagi P, Banerjee R, Basu S, et al. Intravesical antisense therapy for cystitis using TAT-peptide nucleic acid conjugates. Mol Pharm 2006;3(4):398–406.

[72] Lazzeri M, Spinelli M, Beneforti P, et al. Intravesical infusion of resiniferatoxin by a temporary in situ drug delivery system to treat interstitial cystitis: a pilot study. Eur Urol 2004;45(1):98–102.

[73] Miller LJ, Chandler SW, Ippoliti CM. Treatment of cyclophosphamide-induced hemorrhagic cystitis with prostaglandins. Ann Pharmacother 1994;28(5): 590–4.

[74] Saito T, Ikeda Y, Ito E, et al. [Bladder irrigation with prostaglandin E2 in cyclophosphamide-induced hemorrhagic cystitis]. Gan To Kagaku Ryoho 1988;15(1):155–7.

[75] Ippoliti C, Przepiorka D, Mehra R, et al. Intravesicular carboprost for the treatment of hemorrhagic cystitis after marrow transplantation. Urology 1995; 46(6):811–5.

[76] Jeong B, Bae YH, Kim SW. Drug release from biodegradable injectable thermosensitive hydrogel of PEG-PLGA-PEG triblock copolymers. J Control Release 2000;63(1–2):155–63.

[77] Ronneberger B, Kao WJ, Anderson JM, et al. In vivo biocompatibility study of ABA triblock copolymers consisting of poly(L-lactic-co-glycolic acid) A blocks attached to central poly(oxyethylene) B blocks. J Biomed Mater Res 1996;30(1):31–40.

[78] Jeong B, Bae YH, Kim SW. In situ gelation of PEG-PLGA-PEG triblock copolymer aqueous solutions

and degradation thereof. J Biomed Mater Res 2000; 50(2):171–7.

[79] Tyagi P, Li Z, Chancellor M, et al. Sustained intravesical drug delivery using thermosensitive hydrogel. Pharm Res 2004;21(5):832–7.

[80] Parsons CL, Stauffer C, Schmidt JD. Bladder-surface glycosaminoglycans: an efficient mechanism of environmental adaptation. Science 1980;208(4444): 605–7.

[81] Lele BS, Hoffman AS. Mucoadhesive drug carriers based on complexes of poly(acrylic acid) and PEGylated drugs having hydrolysable PEG-anhydride-drug linkages. J Control Release 2000;69(2):237–48.

[82] Genta I, Conti B, Perugini P, et al. Bioadhesive microspheres for ophthalmic administration of acyclovir. J Pharm Pharmacol 1997;49(8):737–42.

[83] Le Visage C, Rioux-Leclercq N, Haller M, et al. Efficacy of paclitaxel released from bio-adhesive polymer microspheres on model superficial bladder cancer. J Urol 2004;171(3):1324–9.

[84] Grabnar I, Bogataj M, Mrhar A. Influence of chitosan and polycarbophil on permeation of a model hydrophilic drug into the urinary bladder wall. Int J Pharm 2003;256(1–2):167–73.

[85] Haas J, Lehr C-M. Developments in the area of bioadhesive drug delivery systems. Expert Opin Biol Ther 2002;2(3):287–98.

[86] Ozturk E, Eroglu M, Ozdemir N, et al. Bioadhesive drug carriers for postoperative chemotherapy in bladder cancer. Adv Exp Med Biol 2004;553:231–42.

[87] Burnett AL, Calvin DC, Chamness SL, et al. Urinary bladder-urethral sphincter dysfunction in mice with targeted disruption of neuronal nitric oxide synthase models idiopathic voiding disorders in humans. Nat Med 1997;3(5):571–4.

[88] Singh SS, Smith KM, Brown DM. Drug retention following intravesical delivery of fluorouracil therapeutic adhesive in C3H mouse bladder. Anticancer Drugs 1996;7(5):507–13.

[89] Chen HH, Le Visage C, Qiu B, et al. MR imaging of biodegradable polymeric microparticles: a potential method of monitoring local drug delivery. Magn Reson Med 2005;53(3):614–20.

[90] Leakakos T, Ji C, Lawson G, et al. Intravesical administration of doxorubicin to swine bladder using magnetically targeted carriers. Cancer Chemother Pharmacol 2003;51(6):445–50.

[91] Ye Z, Chen J, Zhang X, et al. Novel gelatin-adriamycin sustained drug release system for intravesical therapy of bladder cancer. J Tongji Med Univ 2001; 21(2):145–8.

[92] Saito M, Watanabe T, Tabuchi F, et al. Urodynamic effects and safety of modified intravesical oxybutynin chloride in patients with neurogenic detrusor overactivity: 3 years experience. Int J Urol 2004; 11(8):592–6.

[93] Lu Z, Yeh TK, Tsai M, et al. Paclitaxel-loaded gelatin nanoparticles for intravesical bladder cancer therapy. Clin Cancer Res 2004;10(22): 7677–84.

ELSEVIER
SAUNDERS

Urol Clin N Am 33 (2006) 531–537

**UROLOGIC
CLINICS
of North America**

When to Use Antimuscarinics in Men
Who Have Lower Urinary Tract Symptoms

Ji Youl Lee, MD[a], Dae Kyung Kim, MD, PhD[b],
Michael B. Chancellor, MD[c],*

[a]Department of Urology, Catholic University of Korea, School of Medicine, Seoul, Korea
[b]Department of Urology, Eulji University School of Medicine, Daejeon, Korea
[c]Department of Urology, University of Pittsburgh, Suite 700, Kaufmann Building, 3471 Fifth Avenue,
Pittsburgh, PA 15213, USA

Lower urinary tract symptoms (LUTS) in men are believed to most often originate from clinical benign prostate hyperplasia (BPH), the main pathophysiology of which is due to bladder outlet obstruction (BOO) associated with prostatic enlargement. Many patients who have clinical BPH, however, have symptoms of detrusor overactivity (DOA) and symptoms of BOO. In patients who have BOO in addition to DOA, it was reported that storage symptoms persisted in up to 40% of patients even after surgical relief of BOO [1–3]. The clinical presentation of DOA, called overactive bladder (OAB) symptoms, is often similar to that of BOO. Therefore, it is not easy to distinguish between these two conditions or to identify whether the conditions coexist [4].

The initial therapy in men who have LUTS with or without OAB symptoms is most often with α-blockers. It is unfortunate that not all men who have LUTS report relief of their symptoms with α-blockers alone. What is the benefit of adding an antimuscarinic to the treatment regimen in these men who have LUTS and persistent OAB symptoms? This question is addressed in this article. After presenting recent epidemiologic data and the pathophysiologic aspect, the authors review recent, major clinical studies and discuss several issues associated with these questions.

Epidemiology

According to the recent epidemiologic data, the incidence of OAB symptoms is similar throughout all ages in men and women. These data are provided from large-scale epidemiologic OAB studies in the United States [5] and Europe [6].

The European study used direct and telephone interviews across the general population aged 40 years and older [6]. Of the respondents, 16.6% were found to have symptoms suggestive of OAB syndrome using the available definition at the time (> 8 micturitions per 24 hours, urgency or urge incontinence alone or in any combination). Frequency was the most commonly reported symptom (85%), followed by urgency (54%) and urge incontinence (36%). Although the prevalence of urgency and frequency were similar in men and women, urge incontinence was more common in women than in men.

The United States study was conducted with the National Overactive Bladder Evaluation program, a telephone survey designed to assess overall prevalence and burden of OAB (using the current International Continence Society definition) in adults older than 18 years [5]. This study showed that of the respondents, the prevalence of OAB was 16.9% in women and 16.0% in men, increasing with age.

The prevalence of clinical BPH is also known to increase with age. Therefore, it is not surprising that there is considerable overlap of these two conditions. The incidence of DOA associated

* Corresponding author.
  E-mail address: chancellormb@msx.upmc.edu
(M.B. Chancellor).

with BOO has been reported as 30% to 60%. Because of the similarities and the overlap in symptoms of clinical BPH and OAB, it can be difficult to separate these two conditions [4,7–9]. Moreover, because the bladder is an "unreliable witness," it is more difficult to distinguish the pathology responsible for the individual symptoms (Fig. 1).

Pathophysiology

It has been widely believed that storage symptoms such as frequency, nocturia, and urgency in patients who have BOO may be associated with DOA [10]. Based on the histologic evidence of denervation and the significant reduction in cholinergic receptors in the obstructed bladders, denervation supersensitivity has been proposed as a possible mechanism for OAB in BOO [11]. BOO can cause the remodeling of neural pathways associated with voiding reflexes and produce neurogenic bladder dysfunction [12]. In a study of human detrusor tissue from OAB patients, electron microscopic examinations revealed an alteration of intercellular junctions, which had been proposed as a pathway of electrical coupling. These connections would allow the propagation of action potentials and, thus, synchronous contraction throughout the bladder. These changes suggest that partial denervation of the detrusor smooth muscle may be responsible for increased excitability and increased activity to spread between cells, resulting in an uninhibited contraction of the whole detrusor [3,13,14].

The role of free radicals was proposed as another causative factor of DOA in a partial-BOO model [15]. Free radicals are generated from the cyclic ischemia/hypoxia damages in the obstructed bladder. In turn, these reactions, including the generation of free radicals and the disruption of calcium homeostasis, were suggested as causing specific damage to neuronal membranes, sarcoplasmic reticulum, and mitochondria in the cell. DOA may develop as a result of these damages.

A basal release of acetylcholine from non-neuronal (urothelial) and neuronal sources has been demonstrated in isolated human detrusor muscle [16]. It is suggested that this release, which is increased by stretching and by aging, contributes to DOA and OAB by eventually increasing bladder afferent activity during storage. Antimuscarinics may exert their predominant effect during the filling/storage phase, which enables the bladder to increase capacity and to reduce urgency.

In addition, changes of α-adrenergic receptors (α-ARs) with BOO should be considered in the pathophysiology of DOA. The functional role of α-ARs in normal detrusor muscle has not been established [17]. Functional changes of these α-ARs may be associated with BOO and bladder overactivity. The irritative symptoms of BPH and outflow obstruction, which are relieved by α-AR blocker treatment, have been associated with bladder dysfunction due to obstruction. There is evidence that α-ARs are involved in spinal control of sympathetic, somatic (filling), and parasympathetic voiding reflex. The beneficial effects of α-blockers on filling symptoms, which can be obtained even in the absence of outflow obstruction, support the involvement of extravesical—possibly spinal—α-ARs in the pathogenesis of these symptoms (Fig. 2).

The long-term effects of α-blocker administration need to be studied, especially because animal experiments indicate that α-blockers can alter levels of α-AR mRNA in the base of the rat

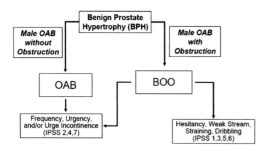

Fig. 1. The symptoms of OAB overlap with those attributed to BOO.

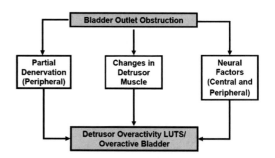

Fig. 2. Potential pathophysiology of DOA in association with male BOO and concomitant LUTS/BPH.

bladder and prostatic urethra, and possibly influence growth of these areas [18].

Clinical study: a series of antimuscarinics in bladder outlet obstruction in men who have detrusor overactivity

The authors recently published their series in the *BJU International* [19] on the role of antimuscarinics in urodynamically verified obstructed men who did and did not have DOA. Based on urodynamic assessment, men who had LUTS were diagnosed with BOO only or with BOO plus DOA symptoms (Fig. 3). Enrollment was restricted to those who had unremarkable results on digital rectal examination, normal urinalysis, prostate-specific antigen (PSA) level less than 6 ng/mL, and postvoid residual volume less than 150 mL. Patients who had neurologic disorders,

a history of genitourinary malignancy or surgery, or history of heart or renal failure were excluded, as were those taking α-blockers, finasteride, or antimuscarinics.

Intervention and outcome

All enrollees received doxazosin at bedtime, at a starting dose of 2 mg. If symptoms had not improved after 1 month, the dose was increased to 4 mg/d for the next 2 months. Men whose symptoms improved after 3 months continued doxazosin monotherapy for a further 3 months. Lack of symptomatic improvement after 3 months of doxazosin monotherapy prompted a switch to combination treatment (once-daily doxazosin plus 2 mg of tolterodine twice daily). Efficacy was assessed as symptomatic improvement; adverse events were monitored (see Fig. 3).

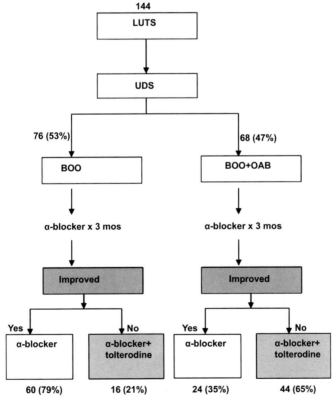

Fig. 3. The study design for patients who have BOO or BOO plus OAB. UDS, pressure/flow urodynamics. (*From* Lee JY, Kim HW, Lee SJ, et al. Comparison of doxazosin with or without tolterodine in men with symptomatic bladder outlet obstruction and an overactive bladder. BJU Int 2004;94(6):817–20; with permission.)

Results

Of 204 potential participants who had BOO, 144 satisfied entry criteria. The 68 subjects (47%) diagnosed with BOO plus DOA were older than the 76 (53%) diagnosed with BOO only (mean 68.5 years versus 63.1 years, $P = .001$). At baseline, men who had BOO plus DOA also reported a higher International Prostate Symptom Score (IPSS): the mean IPSS was 25.2 versus 21.5 ($P = .001$). Urodynamic parameters (other than magnitude of involuntary detrusor contractions) were similar between the two groups, as was the severity of BOO.

Three months of doxazosin treatment at least partially relieved symptoms in 60 of the 76 men (79%) who had BOO only. This initial monotherapy regimen also improved symptoms in 24 of the 68 men (35%) who had BOO plus DOA. Of the 16 patients who had BOO only whose symptoms did not improve after 3 months of doxazosin, 6 (38%) reported improvement following combination treatment with doxazosin plus tolterodine. This combination also afforded symptomatic relief to 32 of the 44 men (73%) who had BOO plus DOA in whom doxazosin alone had been ineffective (Figs. 4 and 5).

Adverse effects of doxazosin were abnormal ejaculation (1.3%), dizziness (2.0%), and postural hypotension (1.3%). Sixteen of the 60 men (27.0%) who received tolterodine reported dry mouth, predominantly of mild or moderate severity. Two men in the combination treatment group experienced temporary acute urinary retention.

Comments

The authors' findings indicate that many men who have BOO also have DOA. Symptoms related to these conditions can be similar, and distinguishing between the two conditions can be difficult based on clinical presentation alone. These results showed that doxazosin—a nonspecific, long-acting α_1-AR antagonist—improves IPSS score by at least 3 points, mainly in those who did not have concomitant DOA. When tolterodine was added to the treatment regimen of those in whom doxazosin was not effective, 6 of the 16 men (38%) improved. Adverse effects were infrequent. The combination of doxazosin and tolterodine might be proposed as a second therapeutic step in men who have BOO but do not respond to α-blockers.

Clinical safety issues of antimuscarinics in bladder outlet obstruction

Many clinicians avoid using antimuscarinics in men because of concerns regarding a potential decrease in detrusor contractility, which could theoretically increase the risk of acute urinary retention. The clinical safety of antimuscarinics in the population of men who have OAB and BOO, however, has been demonstrated in several clinical trials. Abrams [20] reported that of 221 men older than age 40 years who had BOO and OAB and were randomized to 12 weeks of oral treatment with tolterodine (2 mg twice daily) or to placebo, only 1 man in each treatment group experienced temporary acute urinary retention. Moreover, immediate-release tolterodine did not significantly affect urinary flow or detrusor function as assessed by urodynamic evaluation [21].

The authors' study also confirmed the low risk of urinary retention in men who have urodynamically documented BOO when treated with combined doxazosin and tolterodine [19]. Acute

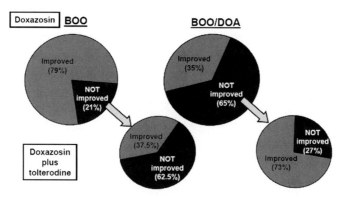

Fig. 4. Clinical improvement rates in each step of treatment in the BOO and BOO/DOA subgroups.

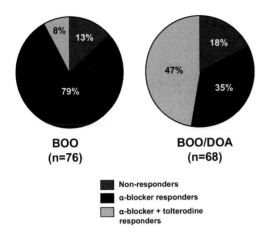

BOO
(n=76)

BOO/DOA
(n=68)

■ Non-responders
■ α-blocker responders
▨ α-blocker + tolterodine
responders

Fig. 5. Overall proportions of responders in the BOO and BOO/DOA subgroups.

urinary retention developed in only 2 of 60 men (3.3%) treated with the combination treatment of doxazosin and tolterodine. The retentions resolved within 48 hours after stoppage of tolterodine in both cases.

In another recent report of combination treatment in men who had OAB coexisting with BOO due to benign prostatic enlargement, the safety and efficacy of doxazosin versus doxazosin plus propiverine were compared [22]. At 8 weeks after treatment, combination treatment with propiverine and doxazosin improved storage symptoms including voiding frequency and urgency and increased patient satisfaction more significantly than treatment with doxazosin alone, but not in nocturia. Although the overall adverse event rates were higher in the combination group, the discontinuation rates due to adverse events were not different between groups. Moreover, propiverine did not affect the urinary flow rate, and no acute urinary retention was observed. These results suggest that antimuscarinics are clinically safe and effective for monotherapy or combination treatment with α-blockers in selected patients who have OAB coexisting with BOO.

Urodynamic study issues: is it necessary in bladder outlet obstruction and overactive bladder?

At the 2004 American Urological Association meeting, Okada and colleagues [23] reported on their series that evaluated the effects of combination treatment with α-blockers and antimuscarinics. This study from Japan is notable for two reasons. First, propiverine, a mixed-function agent

that has antimuscarinic and calcium-blocking effects, was used in combination treatment with a α-blockers. The dual effect of propiverine may help to further decrease uninhibited detrusor contractions, although it may escalate the potential risk of urinary retention. Second, the investigators used purely symptomatic criteria (IPSS subscore) for their patient selection. In this study, no sophisticated urodynamic evaluation was done except uroflowmetry and residual urine measurement.

Of 355 patients who had symptomatic BPH who failed α-blocker treatment for at least 4 weeks, 35 patients who had mainly irritative symptoms (IPSS subscores 2, 4, and $7 > 3$; IPSS subscores 1, 3, and $6 \leq 2$; subscore $5 \leq 3$) were selected for combination treatment. The patients were treated with α-blockers and propiverine for 12 weeks. After treatment, total IPSS decreased from 20.4 to 15.8 ($P < .05$). The IPSS subscores 2, 4, 5 and 7 showed significant improvement, whereas the IPSS subscores 1, 3, and 6 did not change significantly. Maximum flow rate and voided volumes increased from 8.7 to 9.5 mL/s ($P < .05$) and from 98 to 130 mL ($P < .05$), respectively. Postvoiding residual urine volumes did not change significantly. Quality-of-life (QOL) score improved from 4.75 to 3.25 ($P < .05$). No urinary retention was reported. This study suggests that selected patients who have mainly irritative symptoms have favorable responses to combination treatment with α_1-AR blockers and propiverine without increases in obstructive symptoms.

The usefulness of urodynamic studies in men who have symptomatic BOO with or without OAB before antimuscarinics remains highly controversial. Knutson and colleagues [24] reported that 89 of 162 men (55%) who had LUTS had a stable bladder, and 73 (45%) had DOA on cystometry. Although no significant differences were found in serum creatinine, maximum flow rate, postvoiding residual urine volumes, IPSS, and prostate ultrasound volumes, significant differences were found in age, PSA, voided volume, and obstruction grade between the two groups.

In the authors' series previously mentioned [19], 68 of 144 patients (47%) had coexisting DOA according to cystometry, but there was no significant difference between the BOO-only or the BOO plus OAB groups, except for age. Seventy-nine percent of BOO-only patients, however, had symptomatic improvement after taking doxazosin, with a decrease in the IPSS of more than 3 points, but only 35% of the men who had BOO and coexisting OAB had clinical improvement with an α-blocker alone. This result suggests that urodynamic evaluation can help determine whether to start early combination treatment with antimuscarinics.

Quality-of-life issues and the Athanasopoulos and colleagues' study

Although symptom severity may not correlate with perceived bother and effect, the impact of treatment on QOL has always been an important issue when the efficacy of a specific treatment (especially for voiding dysfunction) is evaluated. It is widely accepted that storage symptoms are more bothersome and have a negative impact on patient QOL. In their work at the University of Patras in Greece, Athanasopoulos and associates [25] demonstrated that combination treatment improved QOL in patients who had BOO and concomitant DOA.

In this study, 50 consecutive patients who had urodynamically verified mild or moderate BOO and concomitant DOA were enrolled [25]. After initial treatment with tamsulosin (0.4 mg/d) for 1 week, the patients were randomly allocated into two groups: group 1 received continued tamsulosin only and group 2 received a combination treatment of tamsulosin plus tolterodine (2-mg orally twice daily). After 3 months of treatment, a significant difference was noted in both groups in maximum flow rate and volume at first contraction. Statistically significant improvement in QOL scores, however, was noted only in the patients of group 2. Although 2 patients from group 2 stopped tolterodine due to dry mouth, no acute urinary retention was observed. Tolterodine did not affect the quality of urine flow or residual urine volume. These data suggest that combination treatment is safe and results in a statistically significant improvement in QOL scores.

Antimuscarinic monotherapy in male lower urinary tract symptoms and the Kaplan and colleagues' study

According to a recent study published in the *Journal of Urology* [26], extended-release tolterodine significantly improved lower urinary tract storage symptoms from baseline in men after unsuccessful treatment with α-blocker therapy. Men who have LUTS are often diagnosed as having BPH and initially treated with α-blockers; however, many patients treated with α-blockers report

persistent frequency and urgency of urination. This study is the latest to suggest that tolterodine may be a reasonable therapeutic option in men who have LUTS.

In the open-label, prospective study, Kaplan and colleagues [26] treated 43 men aged 50 years or older with extended-release tolterodine, 4 mg, for 6 months. Inclusion criteria were the confirmation of BPH with digital rectal examination and PSA level plus the termination of α-blocker treatment (duration at least for 1 month) because of adverse events or a lack of efficiency. Mean LUTS, as measured by the American Urological Association symptom score, improved over the 6-month period. Mean daytime urination frequency decreased from 9.8 episodes to 6.3 episodes per day, whereas mean nighttime urination frequency decreased from 4.1 episodes to 2.9 episodes per night. There were no reports of urinary retention.

Although this study was small and lacked of urodynamic verification of obstructive status, the results suggest that antimuscarinic monotherapy can be another favorable option in the management of LUTS secondary to BPH.

Changing the benign prostate hyperplasia and lower urinary tract symptoms market

There is tremendous potential for the United States BPH and LUTS market, considering that only 20% of the affected population was treated in 2005. Comorbidities are common among men 50 years and older due to their numerous health and lifestyle challenges. Erectile dysfunction, OAB, coronary artery disease, and male pattern baldness are highly prevalent comorbidities among patients who have BPH. Antimuscarinics, which are approved for DOA, are likely to help many men who have BPH and LUTS. LUTS may have numerous causes and can occur along with conditions such as BPH, OAB, or others.

Summary

Not all men who have LUTS can be adequately treated with α-blockers alone. Based on objective urodynamic diagnosis, combination treatment can be started early, circumventing the need for an evaluation period of α-blocker monotherapy usually lasting several months. BOO with concomitant DOA appears to be able to safely and accurately be treated with the combination of α-blockers and antimuscarinics.

References

[1] Leppanen MK. A cystometric study of the function of the urinary bladder in prostatic patients. Urol Int 1962;14:226–38.

[2] Price DA, Ramsden PD, Stobbart D. The unstable bladder and prostatectomy. Br J Urol 1980;52(6):529–31.

[3] Brading AF, Turner WH. The unstable bladder: towards a common mechanism. Br J Urol 1994;73(1):3–8.

[4] Blaivas JG. Obstructive uropathy in the male. Urol Clin North Am 1996;23(3):373–84.

[5] Stewart WF, Van Rooyen JB, Cundiff GW, et al. Prevalence and burden of overactive bladder in the United States. World J Urol 2003;20(6):327–36.

[6] Irwin DE, Milsom I, Kopp Z, et al. Impact of overactive bladder symptoms on employment, social interactions and emotional well-being in six European countries. BJU Int 2006;97(1):96–100.

[7] Andersen JT. Detrusor hyperreflexia in benign inravesical obstruction. A cystometric study. J Urol 1976;115(5):532–4.

[8] Andersen JT, Nordling J, Walter S. Prostatism. I. The correlation between symptoms, cystometric and urodynamic findings. Scand J Urol Nephrol 1979;13(3):229–36.

[9] Geirsson G, Fall M, Lindstrom S. Subtypes of overactive bladder in old age. Age Ageing 1993;22(2):125–31.

[10] Blaivas JG. Pathophysiology and differential diagnosis of benign prostatic hypertrophy. Urology 1988;32(6 Suppl):5–11.

[11] Speakman MJ, Brading AF, Gilpin CJ, et al. Bladder outflow obstruction–a cause of denervation supersensitivity. J Urol 1987;138(6):1461–6.

[12] Sutherland RS, Baskin LS, Kogan BA, et al. Neuroanatomical changes in the rat bladder after bladder outlet obstruction. Br J Urol 1998;82(6):895–901.

[13] Brading AF. A myogenic basis for the overactive bladder. Urology 1997;50(6A Suppl):57–67 [discussion: 68–73].

[14] Elbadawi A, Yalla SV, Resnick NM. Structural basis of geriatric voiding dysfunction. III. Detrusor overactivity. J Urol 1993;150(5 Pt 2):1668–80.

[15] Levin RM, Levin SS, Zhao Y, et al. Cellular and molecular aspects of bladder hypertrophy. Eur Urol 1997;32(Suppl 1):15–21.

[16] Andersson KE, Yoshida M. Antimuscarinics and the overactive detrusor—which is the main mechanism of action? Eur Urol 2003;43(1):1–5.

[17] Andersson K. Alpha1-adrenoceptors and bladder function. Eur Urol 1999;36(Suppl 1):96–102.

[18] Yono M, Foster HE Jr, Shin D, et al. Doxazosin-induced up-regulation of alpha 1A-adrenoceptor mRNA in the rat lower urinary tract. Can J Physiol Pharmacol 2004;82(10):872–8.

[19] Lee JY, Kim HW, Lee SJ, et al. Comparison of doxazosin with or without tolterodine in men with symptomatic bladder outlet obstruction and an overactive bladder. BJU Int 2004;94(6):817–20.

[20] Abrams P. Tolterodine therapy in men with bladder outlet obstruction and symptomatic detrusor overactivity is not associated with urinary safety concerns. J Urol 2002;167(Suppl 2002):1048.

[21] Abrams P, Kaplan SA, Millard R. Tolterodine treatment is safe in men with bladder outlet obstruction (BOO) and symptomatic detrusor overactivity (DO). Neurourol Urodyn 2001;20:547–8.

[22] Lee KS, Choo MS, Kim DY, et al. Combination treatment with propiverine hydrochloride plus doxazosin controlled release gastrointestinal therapeutic system formulation for overactive bladder and coexisting benign prostatic obstruction: a prospective, randomized, controlled multicenter study. J Urol 2005;174(4 Pt 1):1334–8.

[23] Okada H, Shrakawa T, Muto S, et al. Propiverine hydrochloride relieves irritative symptoms of benign prostatic hyperplasia. J Urol 2004;(Suppl 171):357.

[24] Knutson T, Edlund C, Fall M, et al. BPH with coexisting overactive bladder dysfunction–an everyday urological dilemma. Neurourol Urodyn 2001;20(3):237–47.

[25] Athanasopoulos A, Gyftopoulos K, Giannitsas K, et al. Combination treatment with an alpha-blocker plus an anticholinergic for bladder outlet obstruction: a prospective, randomized, controlled study. J Urol 2003;169(6):2253–6.

[26] Kaplan SA, Walmsley K, Te AE. Tolterodine extended release attenuates lower urinary tract symptoms in men with benign prostatic hyperplasia. J Urol 2005;174(6):2273–5 [discussion: 2275–76].

ELSEVIER
SAUNDERS

Urol Clin N Am 33 (2006) 539–543

UROLOGIC
CLINICS
of North America

The Promise of β3-adrenoceptor Agonists to Treat the Overactive Bladder

Akira Furuta, MD[a], Catherine A. Thomas, PhD[a], Masahide Higaki, PhD[a], Michael B. Chancellor, MD[a], Naoki Yoshimura, MD, PhD[a], Osamu Yamaguchi, MD, PhD[b],*

[a]Department of Urology, University of Pittsburgh School of Medicine, Suite 700, Kaufmann Building, 3471 Fifth Avenue, Pittsburgh, PA 15213, USA
[b]Department of Urology, Fukushima Medical University School of Medicine, 1 Hikarakigaoka, Fukushima City, 960-1295, Fukushima, Japan

In the detrusor muscle of several mammals including humans, there are β-adrenoceptors (β-ARs) [1–3] whose function may be to mediate relaxation of the detrusor during urine storage [4]. Becauase β-ARs dominate over α-ARs post-junctionally in the bladder [5], noradrenaline relaxes the detrusor through stimulation of β-ARs in the normal condition. β-AR agonists are known to stimulate adenylate cyclase to increase cyclic AMP (cAMP). In turn, cAMP activates protein kinase A (PKA) to mediate the biologic effects. There are two subtypes—β1-AR and β2-AR—that have been identified in the urinary bladder of many species including humans. In most species, the β2-AR subtype has been shown to have an important role in relaxation by way of activation of adenylate cyclase [6–8]. In humans, however, isoproterenol-induced relaxation of detrusor is not blocked by practolol (a selective β1-AR antagonist) or butoxamine (a selective β2-AR antagonist), suggesting that β-ARs in human detrusor are of a different subtype [9,10]. Indeed, a third type of β-AR (β3-AR) has also been implicated in the mediation of metabolic functions such as lipolysis, thermogenesis, antiobesity activity, and motility processes of endogenous catecholamines in the gastrointestinal tract [11,12].

In this article, the authors review the evidence for β3-AR in human detrusor muscle and urothelium and discuss the potential use of β3-AR agonists for the treatment of overactive bladder. In addition, the cAMP-dependent and -independent mechanisms of relaxation by way of β-ARs in rat detrusor muscle, with and without precontraction, are reported [13]. Finally, the consequences of mutation of a β3-AR gene (relating to the pathophysiology of idiopathic detrusor instability) are discussed.

Characterization and function of β3-adrenoceptors in human detrusor and urothelium

The characterization and cloning of a β3-AR gene from the human genomic library [14], mouse genomic library [15], and rat brown adipose complementary DNA library [16] has been accomplished. Thus, instead of using pharmacologic methods or binding assays, the β-AR subtypes can be discriminated by evaluating mRNA encoding the three subtypes. Recently, the expression of β1-, β2-, and β3-AR in mRNA in human detrusor has been reported [17–19]. To determine the relative abundance of β1-AR, β2-AR, and β3-AR in human detrusor, a quantitative analysis of β1-, β2-, and β3-AR mRNAs was performed in bladder tissue from 10 patients (6 men and 4 women, 40–75 years old) who had bladder cancer and underwent radical cystectomy [20]. Using real-time quantitative polymerase chain reaction, based on the TaqMan chemistry system (ABI PRISM 7700 sequence detection system; Perkin-Elmer,

* Corresponding author.
E-mail address: yamaosa@fmu.ac.jp (O. Yamaguchi).

0094-0143/06/$ - see front matter © 2006 Elsevier Inc. All rights reserved.
doi:10.1016/j.ucl.2006.06.014

urologic.theclinics.com

Chiba, Japan), a predominant expression of β_3-AR mRNA was detected in this tissue. Thus, the average number of copies of β-AR mRNA per nanogram of total RNA was 5.46 and 5.27 for the β_1-AR mRNA and β_2-AR mRNA, respectively, compared with approximately 358 for β_3-AR mRNA (Fig. 1). Thus, of the three subtypes of mRNA, 97% was represented by the β_3-AR subtype, and only 1.5% and 1.4% for the β_1-AR and β_2-AR, respectively [20]. If the amount of mRNA subtype reflects the population of receptor protein, then the β_3-AR is the most abundant in human detrusor muscle, suggesting that this subtype mediates detrusor relaxation.

It has been shown that β-AR activation by isoproterenol in rat urothelial cells can trigger production and release of nitric oxide (NO) due to an increase in intracellular Ca^{2+} following activation of the adenylate cyclase pathway in urothelial cells [21]. Recently, the authors identified the presence of β_1-, β_2-, and β_3-AR in bladder mucosa including the urothelium and in the detrusor layer of human bladders (Fig. 2) [22]. Because NO has only minimal relaxing effects on rat bladder smooth muscles [23], it was suggested that NO can decrease overactive bladder by suppressing excitability of the release of transmitters from bladder afferent nerves. Thus, it seems reasonable to assume that information about β-ARs expressed in the human urothelium might be involved in the regulation of bladder sensory functions.

β-adrenoceptors and the cyclic AMP–dependent and –independent mechanisms

The mechanism by which β-AR agonists induce relaxation of smooth muscles is not fully understood, but it is believed that an intracellular pathway for smooth muscle relaxation is activated by cAMP. Activation of β-AR couples by way of G proteins to adenylate cyclase, leading to an increase in intracellular cAMP levels and a subsequent activation of cAMP-dependent PKA [24]. PKA then phosphorylates myosin light chain kinase, which suppresses a calcium-calmodulin–dependent interaction of myosin with actin. The increase in cAMP production also results in attenuation of cytoplasmic Ca^{2+} concentration by removal of Ca^{2+} from cytoplasm. Kobayashi and colleagues [25] showed that the isoproterenol-induced relaxation of guinea pig bladder smooth muscles was mainly mediated by facilitation of calcium-activated K^+ (BK_{Ca}) channels subsequent to the activation of the cAMP/PKA pathway. If BK_{Ca} channels are activated solely by this cAMP-dependent pathway, then an adenylate cyclase inhibitor (SQ22536) would suppress the isoproterenol-induced relaxation to the same extent as a BK_{Ca} channel inhibitor (eg, charybdotoxin and iberiotoxin). Uchida and colleagues' [13] results, however, showed that in high-K^+ precontracted detrusor muscle, the inhibitory effect of SQ22536 on relaxation elicited by isoproterenol was much smaller than by charybdotoxin and iberiotoxin, suggesting that in rat detrusor muscle, BK_{Ca} channels may be activated mainly by means independent of cAMP formation. This study indicates that in noncontracted detrusor muscle, relaxation mediated through β-ARs is achieved solely by cAMP-dependent mechanisms, whereas in KCl precontracted detrusor muscle, cAMP-dependent and cAMP-independent mechanisms by way of BK_{Ca} channels may be involved in β-adrenergic relaxation. Likewise, Petkov and

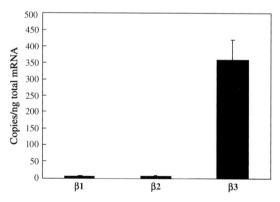

Fig. 1. Distribution of β-adrenoceptor subtype messenger RNA (mRNA) in human detrusor. Data shown are mean $\pm$ SEM (n = 10). (*Adapted from* Yamaguchi O. β3-adrenoceptors in human detrusor muscle. Urology 2002;59(Suppl 5A):26; with permission.)

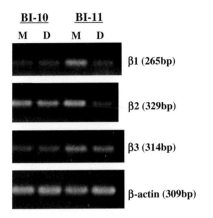

Fig. 2. β-adrenoceptor subtype mRNA in human mucosa (M) and detrusor (D) by reverse transcriptase–polymerase chain reaction.

Nelson [26] showed that β-ARs stimulation activated BK_{Ca} channels by elevating Ca^{2+} influx through voltage-dependent Ca^{2+} channels (VDCC) and by increasing Ca^{2+} sparks. Their data, however, did not support a mechanism involving direct activation of the BK_{Ca} channels by β-ARs because isoproterenol did not activate the BK_{Ca} current when VDCC were inhibited with nifedipine [26].

Therapeutic potential for drugs acting at β₃-adrenoceptors

The in vivo effects of β₃-AR agonists on bladder function have been studied in animal models. Relaxation of rat detrusor muscles is mediated not only by β₂-AR but also by β₃-AR [17,27]. Using cystometry in a conscious rat model of urinary frequency induced by ibotenic acid injection, oral administration of the β₃-AR agonist FK 175 at a dose of 10 mg/kg was shown to increase bladder capacity significantly from 231 μL to 389 μL, with no change of micturition pressure or threshold pressure [17]. Likewise, cystometry in urethane-anesthetized rats showed that compared with other agents (including isoproterenol, verapamil, and atropine), intravenous administration of the β₃-AR agonist CL 316,243 at a dose of 10 mg/kg increased bladder capacity and did not change the residual volume. Of the compounds tested, CL 316,243 also had the weakest cardiovascular side effects as assessed by changes in heart rate and blood pressure [27]. Activation of β₃-AR in the urothelium could have additional relaxant effects on the bladder due to increased release of NO from urothelial cells. Thus the clinical development of β₃-AR agonists for treatment of overactive bladder has been encouraged. Given that activation of β₃-AR on adipocytes (fat cells) leads to lipolysis and an increase in energy use, several rat β₃-receptor-selective agonists that showed antiobesity effects in animal studies were studied in humans as antiobesity agents. It is unfortunate that these studies revealed that any therapeutic benefits derived from these agents were complicated by side effects of tremor and tachycardia, probably mediated by way of β₂-AR and β₁-AR. These studies also indicated that pharmacologic differences existed between the rat and human β₃-receptors. Thus, in future clinical trials for overactive bladder, β₃-AR agonists that are highly selective for the human β₃-AR but not for β₂-AR and β₁-AR are awaited.

Consequences of β₃-adrenoceptor gene mutation

A missense mutation in codon 64 of the β₃-AR gene with a replacement of tryptophan (Trp) to arginine (Arg) occurs with an approximate frequency of 8% to 10% in the white population, 20% in the Japanese population, and 40% in Alaskan Eskimos [28]. This mutation is associated with abdominal obesity, insulin resistance, an increased capacity to gain weight, difficulty in losing weight, and a high body mass index [29–31]. Because activation of the β₃-AR causes a relaxation of detrusor muscle during bladder filling, the authors hypothesized that mutation of the β₃-AR gene may also be involved in idiopathic overactive bladder, leading to an insufficient relaxation of bladder during urine storage, decreasing bladder capacity and favoring unstable contraction.

The authors have therefore begun to explore this possibility by examining whether the Trp 64 Arg mutation of the β₃-AR gene may be a genetic marker for idiopathic detrusor instability. Using hair root samples from 43 patients (41 women and 2 men) who had idiopathic detrusor instability, the authors found that approximately 50% had a β₃-AR gene mutation. Thus, 19 patients had the heterozygous (Trp 64 Arg) mutation, 2 had the homozygous (Arg 64 Arg) mutation, and 22 had the normal gene (Trp 64 Trp). The overall mutation frequency was 49% (21/43) in these patients, which is higher than the overall frequency of 20% to 30% reported in the Japanese population [28]. Although these preliminary results await confirmation from larger-scale studies of patient and control groups, they nevertheless provide support for the hypothesis that dysfunction of β_3-AR may be involved in disorders other than obesity.

Summary

The human β_3-AR appears to be a useful target for the therapy of overactive bladder and other disorders. Differentiating between compounds that have selectivity for human versus animal β_3-AR, however, is an important consideration in the continued study of this receptor. The development of compounds that have high selectivity for the human β_3-AR will not only aid in the production of new therapeutic modalities but also help elucidate the mechanisms of detrusor instability.

References

[1] Morrison LM, Eadie AS, McAlister A, et al. Personality testing in 226 patients with urinary incontinence. Br J Urol 1986;58:387–9.

[2] Morita T, Dohkita S, Kondo S, et al. Cyclic adenosine monophosphate production and contractile response induced by beta-adrenoceptor subtypes in rabbit urinary bladder smooth muscle. Urol Int 1990;45:10–5.

[3] Li JH, Yasay GD, Kau ST. β-Adrenoceptor subtypes in the detrusor of guinea-pig urinary bladder. Pharmacology 1992;44:13–8.

[4] Andersson KE. Pharmacology of lower urinary tract smooth muscles and penile erectile tissues. Pharmacol Rev 1993;45:253–308.

[5] Nomiya M, Yamaguchi O. A quantitative analysis of mRNA expression of $\alpha 1$ and β-adrenoceptor subtypes and their functional roles in human normal and obstructed bladders. J Urol 2003;170:649–53.

[6] Maggi CA, Meli A. Modulation by β-adrenoreceptors of spontaneous contractions of rat urinary bladder. J Auton Pharmacol 1982;2:255–60.

[7] Levin RM, Ruggieri MR, Wein AJ. Identification of receptor subtypes in the rabbit and human urinary bladder by selective radio-ligand binding. J Urol 1988;139:844–8.

[8] Morita T, Ando M, Kihara K, et al. Species differences in cAMP production and contractile response induced by β-adrenoceptor subtypes in urinary bladder smooth muscle. Neurourol Urodyn 1993;12:185–90.

[9] Nergardh A, Boreus LO, Naglo AS. Characterization of the adrenergic beta-receptor in the urinary bladder of man and cat. Acta Pharmacol Toxicol (Copenh) 1977;40:14–21.

[10] Larssen JJ. α- and β-Adrenoceptors in the detrusor muscle and bladder base of the pig and β- adrenoceptors in the detrusor muscle of man. Br J Pharmacol 1979;65:215–22.

[11] Arch JR, Ainsworth AT, Ellis RD, et al. Treatment of obesity with thermogenic β-adrenoceptor agonists: studies on BRL 26830A in rodents. Int J Obes 1984;8(Suppl 1):1–11.

[12] Bond RA, Clarke DE. Agonist and antagonist characterization of a putative adrenoceptor with distinct pharmacological properties from the α- and β-subtypes. Br J Pharmacol 1988;95:723–34.

[13] Uchida H, Shishido K, Nomiya M, et al. Involvement of cyclic AMP-dependent and –independent mechanisms in the relaxation of rat detrusor muscle via β-adrenoceptors. Eur J Pharmacol 2005;518:195–202.

[14] Emorine LJ, Marullo S, Briend-Sutren MM, et al. Molecular characterization of the human β_3-adrenergic receptor. Science 1989;245:1118–21.

[15] Nahmias C, Blin N, Elalouf JM, et al. Molecular characterization of the mouse β_3-adrenergic receptor: relationship with the atypical receptor of adipocytes. EMBO J 1991;10:3721–7.

[16] Granneman JG, Lahners KN, Chaudhry A. Molecular cloning and expression of the rat β_3-adrenergic receptor. Mol Pharmacol 1991;40:895–9.

[17] Fujimura T, Tamura K, Tsutsumi T, et al. Expression and possible functional role of the $\beta 3$-adrenoceptor in human and rat detrusor muscle. J Urol 1999;161:680–5.

[18] Igawa Y, Yamazaki Y, Takeda H, et al. Functional and molecular biological evidence for a possible β_3-adrenoceptor in the human detrusor muscle. Br J Pharmacol 1999;126:819–25.

[19] Takeda M, Obara K, Mizusawa T, et al. Evidence for β_3-adrenoceptor subtypes in relaxation of the human urinary bladder detrusor: analysis by molecular biological and pharmacological methods. J Pharmacol Exp Ther 1999;288:1367–73.

[20] Yamaguchi O. β3-adrenoceptors in human detrusor muscle. Urology 2002;59(Suppl 5A):25–9.

[21] Birder LA, Nealen ML, Kiss S, et al. β-Adrenoceptor agonists stimulate endothelial nitric oxide synthase in rat urinary bladder urothelial cells. J Neurosci 2002;22(18):8063–70.

[22] Thomas CA, Tyagi S, Masuda H, et al. β-adrenoceptor subtype 1, 2 and 3 mRNA are all present in human detrusor muscle and urothelium. J Urol 2005;173:45A.

[23] Andersson KE, Persson K. Nitric oxide synthase and the lower urinary tract: possible implications for physiology and pathophysiology. Scand J Urol Nephrol 1995;(Suppl 175):43–55.

[24] Gilman AG. G proteins: transducers of receptor-generated signals. Annu Rev Biochem 1987;56:615–49.

[25] Kobayashi H, Adachi-Akahane S, Nagao T. Involvement of BK_{Ca} channels in the relaxation of detrusor muscle via β-adrenoceptors. Eur J Pharmaco 2000;404:231–8.

[26] Petkov GV, Nelson MT. Differential regulation of Ca^{2+}-activated K^+ channels by β-adrenoceptors in guinea pig urinary bladder smooth muscle. Am J Physiol Cell Physiol 2005;288:C1255–63.

[27] Takeda H, Yamazaki Y, Akahane M, et al. Role of the β₃-adrenoceptor in urine storage in the rat: comparison between the selective β₃-adrenoceptor agonist, CL316,243, and various smooth muscle relaxants. J Pharmacol Exp Ther 2000;293:939–45.

[28] Arner P, Hoffstedt J. Adrenoceptor genes in human obesity. J Intern Med 1999;245:667–72.

[29] Widen E, Lehto M, Kanninen T, et al. Association of a polymorphism in the β₃-adrenergic-receptor gene with features of the insulin resistance syndrome in Finns. N Engl J Med 1995;333:348–51.

[30] Clement K, Vaisse C, Manning BSJ, et al. Genetic variation in the β₃-adrenergic receptor and an increased capacity to gain weight in patients with morbid obesity. N Engl J Med 1995;333:352–4.

[31] Yoshida T, Sakane N, Umekawa T, et al. Mutation of β₃-adrenergic-receptor gene and response to treatment of obesity. Lancet 1995;346:1433–4.

ELSEVIER
SAUNDERS

Urol Clin N Am 33 (2006) 545–549

UROLOGIC
CLINICS
of North America

Index

Note: Page numbers of article titles are in **boldface** type.

Moving?

Make sure your subscription moves with you!

To notify us of your new address, find your **Clinics Account Number** (located on your mailing label above your name), and contact customer service at:

E-mail: elspcs@elsevier.com

800-654-2452 (subscribers in the U.S. & Canada)
407-345-4000 (subscribers outside of the U.S. & Canada)

Fax number: 407-363-9661

Elsevier Periodicals Customer Service
6277 Sea Harbor Drive
Orlando, FL 32887-4800

*To ensure uninterrupted delivery of your subscription, please notify us at least 4 weeks in advance of move.

United States Postal Service
Statement of Ownership, Management, and Circulation

1. Publication Title		2. Publication Number	3. Filing Date
Urologic Clinics of North America		0 0 0 - 7 1 1 1	9/15/06

4. Issue Frequency	5. Number of Issues Published Annually	6. Annual Subscription Price
Feb, May, Aug, Nov	4	$210.00

7. Complete Mailing Address of Known Office of Publication (Not printer) (Street, city, county, state, and ZIP+4)

Elsevier Inc.
360 Park Avenue South
New York, NY 10010-1710

Contact Person
Sarah Carmichael

Telephone
(215) 239-3681

8. Complete Mailing Address of Headquarters or General Business Office of Publisher (Not printer)

Elsevier Inc., 360 Park Avenue South, New York, NY 10010-1710

9. Full Names and Complete Mailing Addresses of Publisher, Editor, and Managing Editor (Do not leave blank)

Publisher (Name and complete mailing address)

John Schrefer, Elsevier Inc., 1600 John F. Kennedy Blvd., Suite 1800, Philadelphia, PA 19103-2899

Editor (Name and complete mailing address)

Kerry Holland, Elsevier Inc., 1600 John F. Kennedy Blvd., Suite 1800, Philadelphia, PA 19103-2899

Managing Editor (Name and complete mailing address)

Catherine Bewick, Elsevier Inc., 1600 John F. Kennedy Blvd., Suite 1800, Philadelphia, PA 19103-2899

10. Owner (Do not leave blank. If the publication is owned by a corporation, give the name and address of the corporation immediately followed by the names and addresses of all stockholders owning or holding 1 percent or more of the total amount of stock. If not owned by a corporation, give the names and addresses of the individual owners. If owned by a partnership or other unincorporated firm, give its name and address as well as those of each individual owner. If the publication is published by a nonprofit organization, give its name and address.)

Full Name	Complete Mailing Address
Wholly owned subsidiary of	4520 East-West Highway
Reed/Elsevier Inc., US holdings	Bethesda, MD 20814

11. Known Bondholders, Mortgagees, and Other Security Holders Owning or Holding 1 Percent or More of Total Amount of Bonds, Mortgages, or Other Securities. If none, check box ▸ None

Full Name	Complete Mailing Address
N/A	

12. Tax Status (For completion by nonprofit organizations authorized to mail at nonprofit rates) (Check one)
The purpose, function, and nonprofit status of this organization and the exempt status for federal income tax purposes:
☐ Has Not Changed During Preceding 12 Months
☐ Has Changed During Preceding 12 Months (Publisher must submit explanation of change with this statement)

PS Form 3526, October 1999 (See Instructions on Reverse)

---

13. Publication Title	14. Issue Date for Circulation Data Below
Urologic Clinics of North America	August, 2006

15.	Extent and Nature of Circulation		Average No. Copies Each Issue During Preceding 12 Months	No. Copies of Single Issue Published Nearest to Filing Date
a.	Total Number of Copies (Net press run)		5,050	4,800
b. Paid and/or Requested Circulation	(1)	Paid/Requested Outside-County Mail Subscriptions Stated on Form 3541. (Include advertiser's proof and exchange copies)	2,153	1,878
	(2)	Paid In-County Subscriptions Stated on Form 3541 (Include advertiser's proof and exchange copies)		
	(3)	Sales Through Dealers and Carriers, Street Vendors, Counter Sales, and Other Non-USPS Paid Distribution	1,627	1,638
	(4)	Other Classes Mailed Through the USPS		
c.	Total Paid and/or Requested Circulation [Sum of 15b. (1), (2), (3), and (4)] ▸		3,780	3,516
d. Free Distribution by Mail (Samples, complimentary, and other free)	(1)	Outside-County as Stated on Form 3541	124	107
	(2)	In-County as Stated on Form 3541		
	(3)	Other Classes Mailed Through the USPS		
e.	Free Distribution Outside the Mail (Carriers or other means)			
f.	Total Free Distribution (Sum of 15d. and 15e.) ▸		124	107
g.	Total Distribution (Sum of 15c. and 15f) ▸		3,904	3,623
h.	Copies not Distributed		1,146	1,177
i.	Total (Sum of 15g. and h.) ▸		5,050	4,800
j.	Percent Paid and/or Requested Circulation (15c. divided by 15g. times 100)		96.82%	97.05%

16. Publication of Statement of Ownership
Publication required. Will be printed in the November 2006 issue of this publication. ☐ Publication not required

17. Signature and Title of Editor, Publisher, Business Manager, or Owner

[signature]
Joseph Patanici – Executive Director of Subscription Services

Date
9/15/06

I certify that all information furnished on this form is true and complete. I understand that anyone who furnishes false or misleading information on this form or who omits material or information requested on the form may be subject to criminal sanctions (including fines and imprisonment) and/or civil sanctions (including civil penalties).

Instructions to Publishers

1. Complete and file one copy of this form with your postmaster annually on or before October 1. Keep a copy of the completed form for your records.
2. In cases where the stockholder or security holder is a trustee, include in items 10 and 11 the name of the person or corporation for whom the trustee is acting. Also include the names and addresses of individuals who are stockholders who own or hold 1 percent or more of the total amount of bonds, mortgages, or other securities of the publishing corporation. In item 11, if none, check the box. Use blank sheets if more space is required.
3. Be sure to furnish all circulation information called for in item 15. Free circulation must be shown in items 15d, e, and f.
4. Item 15h., Copies not Distributed, must include (1) newsstand copies originally stated on Form 3541, and returned to the publisher, (2) estimated returns from news agents, and (3), copies for office use, leftovers, spoiled, and all other copies not distributed.
5. If the publication had Periodicals authorization as a general or requester publication, this Statement of Ownership, Management, and Circulation must be published; it must be printed in any issue in October or, if the publication is not published during October, the first issue printed after October.
6. In item 16, indicate the date of the issue in which this Statement of Ownership will be published.
7. Item 17 must be signed.

Failure to file or publish a statement of ownership may lead to suspension of Periodicals authorization.

PS Form 3526, October 1999 (Reverse)